*To Die For*

ALSO BY CAROL LEE

*Crooked Angels*
*The Ostrich Position*
*Friday's Child*
*The Blind Side of Eden*
*Talking Tough*
*Good Grief*

# To Die For

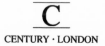

*Carol Lee*

C
CENTURY · LONDON

Published by Century in 2004

5 7 9 10 8 6 4

First published in the United Kingdom in 2004 by Century
The Random House Group Limited
20 Vauxhall Bridge Road, London SW1V 2SA

Random House Australia (Pty) Limited
20 Alfred Street, Milsons Point, Sydney,
New South Wales 2061, Australia

Random House New Zealand Limited
18 Poland Road, Glenfield,
Auckland 10, New Zealand

Random House South Africa (Pty) Limited
Endulini, 5a Jubilee Road, Parktown 2193, South Africa

The Random House Group Limited Reg. No. 954009

www.randomhouse.co.uk

A CIP catalogue record for this book
is available from the British Library

Papers used by Random House are
natural, recyclable products made from wood grown in
sustainable forests. The manufacturing processes conform to
the environmental regulations of the country of origin

ISBN 0 7126 62693

Typeset by Palimpsest Book Production Ltd, Polmont, Stirlingshire
Printed and bound in Great Britain by
Mackays of Chatham PLC

*To 'Emma'*

# *Acknowledgements*

My thanks and appreciation to Gillian McCredie, John Gleisner, Dr Adrienne Key, Dr Eric Johnson-Sabine, Julia Fabricius, Laura Longrigg and Hannah Black for their contributions to this book.

My love and thanks to Jason Williams and my brother, Chris, for practical help and moral support as I wrote it.

# Contents

# *Preface*

This is the story of my god-daughter, Emma's, battle with anorexia and bulimia which began a few weeks after her fifteenth birthday and which lasted at its fiercest for around five years.

Over this span, in the acute part of her illness, Emma's weight went from just over five and a half to almost fourteen stone three times, in three long loops. But an invisible see-saw was swinging inside her from long before.

Anorexia has shadowed much of Emma's life and although her fight with her illness was successful, it has taken years after leaving hospital for the final time for her to feel secure in her recovery.

The account of that time, and what it took to rescue her, are told in the following pages.

NB Many sufferers of anorexia use Body Mass Index (BMI) to measure the progress of their illness.

Emma did not, but her BMI dropped to a severely low 13 in the early stages of her illness and was 31, within the 'obese' range, when she was at her heaviest.

The average BMI for a woman is 19–24.

# *Introduction*

In writing this, I am struck by how many versions of a 'true' story there are depending on where you are standing.

The truth about someone suffering from anorexia is especially difficult to tell because you are almost dealing with a multi-personality – but not quite.

What you are actually dealing with is a multi-age scenario. A person ill with anorexia will fluctuate between a nine and a twenty-year-old and beyond. Emma sometimes spoke to me in the aggressive tones of an arrogant forty-year-old as she sought to overpower and demean me.

So it is not only the sufferer's physical size or weight which is an issue, and which dominates her closed world, it is her age too.

It involves the considerable task, for the helper, not of *who* you are speaking to at any given time, but how old he or she is.

But I was on to Emma by the time I had spotted this, on to something which was invaluable to me in the task of trying to help her: At times she did not so much need looking after as being found out. For she lived a shadowy interior life which bore little relation to the world where I was standing. She needed someone to know this, to know what she was up to, where she was hiding and why.

'Deception' is the word I most associate with anorexia and the treachery which comes from falsehood. The illness appears inviting. It would seem to offer something to those unwary or unlucky enough to suffer from it – friendship, a get-out or a haven – when, in fact, it is a trap.

Emma lived in this trap, in the place she called anorexia, with its 'cold hallways' and 'white walls', for a number of years until, finally, at the age of nineteen, and in hospital for the last time, she called me in.

Battle commenced, anorexia on one side, me on the other. But where was Emma? She switched sides, sometimes allowing herself to be freed a little, and sometimes returning to what she had come to know best.

During these latter times, she would seek to ensnare *me*, her ways of doing it as numerous as the holds the illness had over her. In this fashion, anorexia did many things to both of us.

This is a detective story of a kind. Much of the evidence is contained in two separate sets of diaries written by Emma and by me.

My own came into being for a number of reasons, not least of which was that, after years of silence, Emma began to talk at last about her illness, and I wanted to catch, to record, her words as faithfully as possible.

I started keeping notes of my weekly visits to the Specialist Unit where Emma was hospitalised: how she was; any change in her mood or surroundings; what we said to each other. It seemed wrong to do this behind her back, so I told her about it.

We agreed she should keep diaries too. And I bought her two exercise books with an array of pens, coloured stick-on dots and stars, labels, etc. so she could decorate them if she wished, make them her own.

Keeping our diaries separate was crucial. In her 'young' biddable moments she might have let me read bits of hers, had I asked. And much of what was in them would have taken me so off-track, so far into the wasteland where she was putting up signposts pointing both ways – Life and Death – I would have got lost beyond finding and been of no help to her.

Another reason I kept detailed diaries was to have something to rely on, to hold on to from day to day. As a non-expert with no medical experience, I needed them to give me reference points, signposts to gauge progress, find clues, and a way of trying to understand patterns. They helped me when I got lost, as I did, in the confusing morass of her illness.

Emma did not ask to see my notes and I would not have

let her, for I had treacherous intentions from her point of view, the wish that she should live.

I believe my notes were kept, too, because the outcome of her illness was never certain. I feared, at times, she would die. And if she did, it seemed I had nothing of her, for she was not my daughter.

With my note-keeping, I perhaps wanted something I could remember her by, that might help me understand Emma after death, even. Make her whole. Keep her with me.

For a difficult emotion stalked much of my time with Emma. I was angry with her as she was with me for trying to rescue her. We had many battles.

But had I surrendered to her, we might not be where we are now with Emma, a caring and bright twenty-five-year-old, making her own way. My anger was as necessary as hers. As was the trust I had in her from when she was a toddler.

I am immensely grateful for the trust she has placed in me.

NB to protect people's identities, names have been changed – except those of medical experts.
The entries from Emma's diaries are reproduced as she has written them.

# Chapter One

🦆

## Catching the Words

How things look – appearance, colour, brightness and shade – are important to this story and, standing on the steps waiting to visit Emma, the first thing that strikes me is the view.

From here, the hospital is like an army barracks. Anonymous low brick buildings, a confusing one-way system which sends you away from where you want to go. Heavy speed bumps. No people to be seen.

The Eating Disorders Unit is at the back, away from the main gates overlooking what looks like a goods yard: hundreds of stacked wire crates and, behind them, a couple of chimney stacks, one emitting smoke.

May 1998. Spring you would think, but it is grey and chill from the weather turning back to winter again, and I am cold from waiting when, at last, a buzzer lets me in.

\* \* \*

Relief inside. Warmth, colour, prints on the walls, comfortable furniture, open space. At the reception desk I am told where her room is and, turning a corner, walk towards the closed door – and then stop.

It is more than six months since I last saw her, alone at her parents' house. Silence since then. During the years of her illness, she has a habit of locking me out, keeping me at a distance.

My suggestions that we meet, that she come to my place, we go for a walk, or to a film together, have been ignored. So I have let her be, my concern to let her have her own life, vying with a wish not to allow her to turn her back on me.

But she has rung, extraordinary in itself, to say she is ill, in hospital again, and wishing to see me.

What to do, then, about the door, not even the tiniest bit ajar?

If I knock and she keeps me waiting, or 'doesn't hear', how will that affect my chance of helping her this time?

So, taking a deep breath, stepping forward, I tap, call her name, and, giving her no time to stall, open the door a moment or two later.

'Emma, it's me, Carol,' I say, stepping into the room.

It is modern, well designed: wall-lights; mirrors; cards; belongings; and the stuffed toys she likes so much scattered round. There is a single bed with a pretty cover, wash-basin, drawers, a cupboard.

Standing the other side of the bed, side on, the change

in her is shocking. Many stones dropped since the last time we met, more than five as it turns out, from around eleven and a half to six stone.

Wearing a black, long-sleeved top and dark blue jeans, both loose and hanging on her, she is stooped, listless, but edgy too. She looks dirty. Her usually golden-brown hair is as long as I've seen it, mid-way down her back, dark and matted from sweat and grease.

Her skin is grey, her expression guarded, defensive, her eyes avoiding mine and, as usual, she waits for me to say something, to make the first move.

I hesitate. We have been here before with her illness so many times: me making the running, my wish to 'fill her up' with warmth, affection and a love of being alive; her standing back.

I sense this time will have to be different. She will be twenty in September. This may be her last chance.
Hospital resources are not limitless and this is the third of what seem to have been the unstoppable loops she has gone through.

Each, taking around eighteen months, is driven by something in her I have learned to mistrust – euphoria. High, drunk on it, initially she eats and eats, drives her weight up from a standard nine to ten stone (for her medium height and build) until, at around fourteen she stays, hovering, for a number of months.

At this weight she is big for someone of just over five foot six, but not unattractive. Far from it. She gains weight evenly, has a lovely face and her clear fair skin glows.

Maintaining it for a while, she is seemingly impervious to the outside world, needing no one, barely phoning me. Her extra weight seems to act as a defence for her in these heavy times, her bigness shielding her. Then something happens and, in response to a hidden switch or trigger, she starts, suddenly, to reject food.

In a reverse process of the building up, the piling on, she dives and dives. Gathering speed, pounds, stones falling away, she hurtles back past her mid-point, the safe place of a medium weight.

Numbers, I will learn in this time of visiting, are a problem for her and they blur as she flashes past the figures on the scales on a steep downward path.

Somewhere around five and a half stone or so she crashes, ends up on a hospital ward, as she is now, gone too far for normal functioning or for safety. Too weak to cope.

'Do you want a cuddle?' I ask, but standing where I am, holding my ground. She softens then, straight away, and moves towards me with the warm smile I know so well from her childhood.

With her head on my shoulder, arms draped loosely behind me, gently I hold her and her bones appal me. Her smell, too, is difficult to bear, her hair especially. As if it has not been washed for many weeks, it, and she smell of staleness, sweat and the sourness of fear and neglect.

There is only one chair – no place for us to sit side by side – and I move to the single bed. Propping up pillows at the headboard end, I sit lengthways with my back to it. Emma drapes herself round me, face turned to one side, head under my chin, legs over mine, feet touching.

Over the next few weeks we will spend a lot of time like this. I will enter the room guardedly, sit on the chair for a while, perhaps. Then, when I think it is all right, ask if she wants to be cuddled. She always does, but I always have to ask.

We will then move to the bed and, folding herself over me, she will settle herself down and talk.

Listening attentively, holding her, I have a problem. As the words pour from her, I fear forgetting them, not remembering *exactly* what she says, or not remembering enough. Forgetting things that might seem trivial or irrelevant, but which could be important bits or connections. And with Emma, I need to remember precisely, for in the many arguments which follow she will tax me if I get her words even slightly wrong:

'I never said that.'

I need to remember for another reason: in the years of her illness so far, more than four at this point, she has not said anything about it – at all. She has remained silent, as if blithely assuming the colossal changes in her will not be noticed or challenged.

My early attempts to talk to her, in her first bout of

illness, were met, swiftly, by her shutting me out, not seeing me – until I was called to a hospital bed. Although not, the first two times, by her.

She seemed to expect her dramatic weight gains and sudden dangerous crashes would go unremarked by those around her, and she would not tolerate intrusion.

This time, though, she has asked for me, and it is with great urgency, therefore, that I try to capture how she is and what she has to say.

Arriving home that first night, my head full, I go straight to the computer to off-load.

Emma. May 1998:

> *There's a picture of her, like a bubble in my head, standing, lost in her clothes, in a small room . . .*
>
> *She wants me to visit her every week, says she's been feeling terrible, but thinks she can get better – with my help. She wants us to make a plan for her recovery.*

But, by the time I begin these notes, Emma has recorded her time with anorexia long since. She has written thousands of words in diaries she does not, at this stage, tell me about. She will show me a few pages – soon – and that will be all until her illness is over.

In an entry in March she writes of struggling with two Emmas inside her and speaks to them in her head. One is 'Baby Emma' who does and does not deserve protection, for she is not always an innocent, but sometimes a manipulative, child.

The other is older, the Emma who is more than nineteen, and who decides, ruthlessly at times, to down the child and starve them both.

Emma knows she is both:

> *I want to destroy you, not dry your baby tears and*
> *hold your hand*
> *but we're the same person – why won't you protect*
> *me instead of picking on me?*
> *You don't deserve my protection*
> *why not*
> *Because I hate you*
> *You are me*
> *No I'm not*

The 'I's in 'I hate you' and 'No I'm not' are like big black sticks, twice the size of the other letters, and are almost the only time, for a year or more, when Emma uses a capital letter for herself. Otherwise her place, in her writing, is a small 'i'.

ð

# READING TO EMMA

I first came across Baby Emma a long time ago. By the time she calls me to her hospital room I have known Emma for nearly seventeen years and have a vantage-point on her life. I know her better, I believe, than anybody else, which makes me both valuable to her and a threat.

Emma and I met one afternoon in a London pub – and she adopted me on the spot.
It was that way round.
Sitting at a table by myself for an end-of-week lunch, I saw her for the first time, crossing the pub floor towards me. Between ages, someone more than a toddler and a little less than a small girl, she was, as it turns out, exactly two and three-quarters years old.

Heading in my direction with a heavy glass of lemonade carried tightly in both hands, I watched her be careful not to spill it. Slowly putting it down on the table in front of me, she then climbed up onto the stool opposite, sat down and stared at me.

She had – has – beautiful grey-green eyes, golden-brown hair and a lovely fair skin and that day, I realise, seemed 'old' as well as young, unabashed by me, a stranger, and prepared to hold her ground.

After rather a long time of her unswerving – and silent – scrutiny, I was uncomfortable.

'Do you want some baked beans and mashed potatoes in there?' I asked, nodding from the pub grub on my plate to the soggy half-eaten crisps floating around at the top of her glass.

'You're silly,' she said flatly, her face serious.

'Well, I think you're right about that,' I replied, with a mock sigh and a smile.

'I'm silly, too, sometimes,' she said, scrunching up her shoulders and leaning towards me.

So, that was it.

'Will you read to me?' she asked, head on one side, a moment or two later.

Her obvious delight when I nodded yes was followed by a speedy trip back to the bar. Definitely child-like now, she hoisted herself up again, onto a tall stool this time and, helped by a fair woman behind the counter – her mother, by their close resemblance – brought a cloth bag back for me to open.

This bag was important, Emma's back-pack, or knap-sack as I called it. It was pretty and small, more a Dick

Whittington bag of dreams than a seriously practical affair. Inside was a child's array of colouring pencils, toys and some books.

The bag came to the bar every day with Emma and her mother, Colleen, who had just begun to work lunch-times at the pub. From her position behind the counter, she had checked me out, making sure her daughter was safe in my hands. She and I began to talk. She hoped Emma wasn't being a nuisance, she said.

No, not at all.

Home from home for both of us, the pub gave Colleen part-time work while she retrieved her life, her husband having left her with no money to go back abroad. It gave me a break from my work, writing at home.

So it was that this Friday lunch-time in June was the first of many weekly read-ins at the pub, which soon extended, during the summer, to trips over the road to the small open space of a park opposite to explore and play.

Like all children, Emma loved stories and she was also canny, soon discovering this was no run-of-the-mill grown-up she had taken up with.

Perhaps it was my willingness to join in the jumping about, pretend games she made up which attracted Emma. Or had her antennae picked up something else?

There is a habit of story-telling in our large Welsh family. Oral tradition, if you like, and with nineteen of us first cousins, most with children, and some of those with children too, plenty of it.

Plenty of chance to practice as well, my house sometimes home to an array of under-fives while their mothers,
up from the country, went out to shop. How much was
*Emma* reading *me* I wonder years later.

Whatever, I was sussed and the books she brought with
her were soon left in the bag.

'Not from there,' she would say, patting the bag closed
as we got to 'tell me a story' time: 'one of *your* stories. *You*
tell me, one from your head.'

So, sitting on a bench, or at the edge of the flower beds
on the grass, impromptu stories were invented: a baby
umbrella which liked the rain; a deer who did not; talking
cutlery which got told off for making too much noise in
the kitchen; and chattering mice at the pub over the road.

Where do stories live, we wondered and where would
we look for some? In trees, or under bushes? And what
about stones? How many stories would we find under them
if we looked?

It went on like this during that summer: stories and games
in the park; time spent looking in shop windows, exploring
the locality; chats along the street, her hand in mine.
Pals then.

'Do you know,' she would say to me, testing her big, self-
important voice, 'that fairies live *everywhere*?'

'Really,' I would respond. 'Well, I suppose it doesn't
surprise me now I think about it. They do get around,
these fairies.'

Emma's appetite for language: words; phrases; emphases

– which she was *particularly* fond of – was endearing and I enjoyed seeing her physically grappling with her growing command of speech: getting on top of it; jumping up and down; wrestling it to the ground.

Tripping up over a big word, sometimes, she would look to me for assistance, and, as I silently mouthed it for her, she would, in the next breath, snaffle it up, pummel it into shape and push it into a long sentence all of her own. A skip and a hop, a satisfied: 'Well, that's another one in the bag', and on, with barely a pause, to the next.

Emma had a good ear for the weight and balance of language and paid attention not only to what was said, but to how I said it. On our next lunch-time visit, she would play words and sentences back to me: arm and leg movements too.

'Isn't it amazing,' she said one day, shoulders forward, foot pushed firmly into the ground, 'Teddy didn't want any food at all yesterday.'

'I am surprised. Why do you think that was?'

'Well, it might have been because he couldn't find his medicine bottle . . .'

We shared jokes, Emma and me, and a repertoire of how to cope with the rest of the world when it was annoying us.

With her love of Winnie the Pooh, many an adult was consigned to an imaginary drop down a heffalump hole, both of us deciding when to let him or her out. Were we going to be kind-hearted, on this occasion? After all, this grown-up had some good points. Or were we going to leave her down there a bit longer?

Meanwhile, Colleen and I chatted. In her late twenties, an American waiting for British citizenship, she was reserved until you got to know her and a reluctant barmaid.

Grateful for her daughter to be happily occupied and playing outside. 'You're good with children,' she said to me, one day, with one of her sudden wide smiles.

'I'm used to them,' was my reply.

Emma's third birthday, in September, was celebrated with cards, presents and cakes in the pub and, as she entered her fourth year, some lively and leading questions:

'Why do you only come and see me on Fridays?'

'Because I'm working the rest of the week.'

'Why don't you come and live with Mummy and me?'

'Because I have a house of my own I like living in.'

And, then, the biggee:

'When can I come and see where you live?'

As a writer interviewing hundreds of people over the years, seldom had I, myself, been so swift in pinning someone down. And she was waiting. Looking at me intently, her body still.

'We'll have to talk to your mummy about that, won't we?'

A race to the bar and Emma's excited voice: 'Mummy, Mummy, can I go to Carol's house?'

Seeing Emma for an hour or so on a Friday was enjoyable and, unlike assorted cousins passing through, consistent. I looked forward to our time together, to the changes in her, week by week, and having a break, too, from the heavy demands of work: of writing a newspaper column and, always, the on-going research for a new book. Her coming to my house was different, though, more intimate – and involved.

Over the years which followed, I was told I was not the first grown-up Emma had sought out at the pub for reading duties, just the most willing. But her regular bar days were soon to be over as Colleen gained a British passport and the right to take up a proper job.

We discovered we lived near each other, me in a terraced house and Colleen and Emma in a council flat less than a mile away, with a big park in between.

So, Emma's visits to my home began. And, as she went to nursery, then primary school, the park with its childrens' playground, paddling pool, ponds and open spaces became the place where her imagination grew.

Our playing field.

# Chapter Three

~§

## A GAP IN THE DOOR

The Unit where Emma is housed as a nineteen-year-old is dedicated to the treatment of anorexia. It specialises in researching and treating eating disorders and is geared, therefore, to providing a recovery programme for people like Emma. Attached to a north London hospital, people who stay there are confined to the premises. Locked in.

They are free to move within the Unit itself, a small, self-contained annexe, but they have to ask permission to go out, to make phonecalls and to see people. This is part of a series of inducements and restrictions which patients who go on the recovery programme are expected to accept.

During these early weeks, Emma is allowed only one visitor, and only one visit, a week. She has asked for me, the person, over the years, who has seen through her defences and acknowledged her difficulties.

I sit in the chair to begin with, holding her white teddy which was on the seat before me. Emma shuffles or prowls round the small space. Looking iller than she did last week, she tells me things are bad and shows me the razor cuts she has made, her self-mutilation.

On her arms, wrist, thighs, they surprise, rather than shock, me. So fine and delicate. Less than an inch long, white lines on her skin, fresh, clean among its pallor. Decorative almost. Not wounds. More like adornments.

I say nothing. Instead, run my finger over the smooth markings on her arms. No bumps or joins. Old then, these blood-lettings? Or done with the kind of precision a crafts-man would use. Meticulous. Seamless.

Still I am silent. If these cuts are display not distress, they are a trap, and I must not fall in.

I have learned to be wary of Emma's traps and will rue, on occasion, the shared games of her young childhood as, these years on, I, myself, get lured towards a series of deep heffalump-size holes in the ground.

Her voice husky, a croak at times, we begin to discuss my visits, how we might get her well again, how I might help. She wants me to visit her once a week, she says, to be someone she can look forward to seeing, to be a link with the world outside, and to help her to rejoin it.

Tacitly, we both know that, in a sense, she wants me as a witness. Someone who knows her, a stable person in her moving landscape.

She asks me to take some pictures of her, says she has

a black and white film in her camera, and will I photograph her as she is now. To remind her, she says.

I imagine she means 'before and after', that she will use these pictures to help her get better, measure her progress. Or not.

As it turns out, the pictures are ammunition for her illness, evidence of how reassuringly thin she is, proof that the food she has begun to eat in the last few weeks has left no mark on her, no 'bad' bulge on her skeletal frame. But I do not know this yet.

Instead, I pick up the camera and, through the lens, see a picture – disturbing, arresting – of a girl a little above starvation weight: skull, collar bones, wrists on display, hips jutting. It feels wrong, ghoulish even, to click the shutter, but I do.

Sitting down again on the chair, Emma on the bed opposite facing me, she produces from her locker a hand-made diary: decorated cardboard cover; cut-out pages, only a few written on; all held together by knotted white string. Opening it at a particular page, she hands it to me along with a separate folded sheet – a poem – and waits for me to read.

> what if i die
> before i've made up my mind
> whether or not i want
> to live?
> *I and now i lay me down to sleep*

> *pray my heart is not too weak*
> *to let me live just one more day*
> *in case my hatred blows away!*

Turning to the diary entry, it is from a month earlier and is headed in her neat handwriting and underlined as follows:

> <u>*Wednesday 8th April 1998*</u>
> *i don't want any food to stay inside me and i want to lose weight. i want to weigh lighter than ever before, but i don't want my heart to stop. i don't want to be frightened to go to sleep at night in case i don't wake up again.*

She then writes of the spur for this heart-stopping fear: the death on the Unit a short while earlier of a girl called Katherine – from heart failure.

In the next year or so I will learn that heart muscles are weakened during prolonged bouts of starvation and, while they recover in most people, in some they do not.

> *Katherine and I were getting worse together. Like 2 cars in a game of chicken, seeing who will swerve first – Katherine's car sailed over the cliff, and i'm still heading for it. The game <u>should</u> be over now . . .*
> *Now Katherine is dead. i can't bear the thought*

*of ending up like her, but i can't bear the thought
of not.*

Before these entries, in March, Emma writes of two fears:
one, of a heart attack; the other, of how much of other
people she has taken into herself, swallowed whole. She
writes of imitating the habits of friends at school, and of
them doing the same with her, but who is she if she has
copied other people? How much is she herself?

*i hate the way i adopt other people's mannerisms
and patterns of speech . . . i feel like a parasite
– what would i be like if i just closed myself off
from everyone?*

But she does not do this with Katherine:

*i'm furious with Katherine for dying. She did it,
went all the way – the 'best' anorexic. She beat me
. . . And i hate her for robbing me of that . . .
   If Katherine had not died then i never would
have paused to question the tightness in my chest
and of my breath, never would have wondered why
waking up each morning was such an immense struggle, and i never ever no way not-in-a-million years
EVER would have agreed to come back into hospital. Which is how i know that if Katherine hadn't
died then i would have.*

So this is who I am visiting, whom I have known since childhood, a big-little girl who is huge with deathly intentions, and so small she does not allow herself, in her own diaries, as a capital 'I'. The jigsaw pieces of Emma's anorexia will be difficult for me to fit together over the next eighteen months of seeing her regularly, both in hospital and as a day-patient when she leaves. There is so much thrown at me.

Nor can I easily explain to friends and other people who ask after her that as well as seeing me, she tries, mightily, to lock me out. Since becoming ill, she has stood on the other side of the door to anorexia, pushing hard against it, keeping me firmly, resolutely, on the other side. Something in her wants this more than me, more than anything or anyone.

Across from me she looks crumpled, wretched, shoulders collapsed, hair fallen round her face. Reaching for her, I find she is bathed in sweat. This is what it has cost her, letting me this far in.

A while later, as I leave, I ask if she wants the door to her room left open or closed.

'Open,' she says – and I leave it as it was when I arrived. Looking closed from the end of the corridor, near to it was, almost imperceptibly, a fraction ajar.

# Chapter Four

❦

## Play-Time

Picking up Emma, as a four-year-old, from her home for her first visit to my place, she had been ready, waiting, for an hour, asking her mother, time and again, how long it would be before I came to fetch her.

Knapsack on her back, she was out the door and down two flights of stairs, Colleen and I exchanging hurried helloes and goodbyes as I dashed after her.

Waiting on the pavement by the car, Emma was serious, as well as excited, as if what we were doing was important. A few minutes later, walking round my home, going in every room in the three-storey building, she was quiet. The space was big for her, I realised: high ceilings; large bay windows. Would she be subdued by it, cowed even?

But Emma had made up her mind long since about where I lived and set about claiming it. In the downstairs living room with its French windows leading onto a walled back garden, cushions were fetched to put on the floor, chairs moved, pencils and a colouring book laid out on the table.

I knew Emma would find my place very different from hers. Colour, mainly, as well as space, not only in cushions and curtains, but in other objects: vases; pictures on the walls; and the variegated spines of hundreds of books.

The block of flats where Emma lived seemed bleak by comparison: stairways smelling of stale food; and, inside, where she and Colleen lived, few ornaments, pictures or books. I hoped Emma would enjoy the change in her visits to me, and Colleen, too with some time to herself, away from the demands of a young child.

Over the next few years Emma's regular stays came in three distinct sizes. There was small: an afternoon or after school visit.

Medium was an overnight, Emma plus knapsack awaiting collection from her place on a Saturday afternoon, me on foot or in the car.

Her favourite was the big one: two whole nights. Collection on Friday evening, Emma turning around on the spot in my hallway, giddy with delight, pretending to fall over with happiness. A whole weekend before us, too long to see the end of.

After a while I kept this time just for Emma. Initially, a friend might drop round, or a neighbour's child came to play. Company for her, I thought, someone her own age. But no.

'Who's your favourite child?' she asked one day.

I hesitated. As well as visitors from Wales, a small boy up the road chatted to me regularly over the garden gate, and there were three boys next door.

'You're my favourite girl,' I replied.

We had a problem though: Emma did not like walking. As a three-year-old Colleen had asked me not to give in to her pleas to be picked up a lot.

'She's not a baby any more,' she had said.

So, in our gentle early walks near the pub and in the small park over the road, I had not given in to Emma's wish to be carried. I found it difficult sometimes, her standing on the pavement arms up, saying she was tired, me crouching beside her to encourage her on a little.

She had taken it well, I thought, responded to my cajoling. But as she became four and five, bigger and more capable you would have supposed, her resistance to walking did not go away.

'I don't like it here,' she threw at me bad-temperedly one fine Saturday morning on a trip out to Taplow, near Maidenhead, to walk through the woods down to the river.

We had just seen a tawny owl, wings spread, flying low through the trees, and a fox had stopped a few minutes earlier, clearly visible on the path ahead of us, before veering away as it caught our scent.

'I want to watch TV,' Emma declared.

Physically, Emma was a well-built child. Not fat. Sturdy is the best word to describe her. She was appealing with her large eyes, lovely skin and ever-present seriousness.

Not a chocolate-box girl, but a child with a great deal of character: determination, or stubborness, included. We shared these characteristics, and in arguments later on, during her illness, would be a match for each other.

For now, in her young childhood, I accepted Emma's moods and habits and she, too, put up with mine. There were clear rules in my house which she was expected to go along with. She had a set bed-time, meals were eaten at the table, not in front of the TV, and TV-watching was rationed.

The latter she found especially hard and it took her a long time not to be sulky when it was switched off.

I was determined, though, to wean her away from it. Sitting in the middle of the floor, too near to the screen, shoulders scrunched up, head forward, she would watch for hours if I let her, oblivious to a sunny day outside or children's voices from the street.

For my part of the bargain, I was consistent. I was never late picking her up and kept my promises.

If I agreed, in a weak moment, to let her spin out our Sunday afternoon by agreeing to take her home via the hut in the park, then the hut it was. One of her favourites, a small round wooden place at the edge of the children's playground where we played cooking.

The game was the same, as I remember: her in charge of the oven, and always a crisis or two in the making.

'Do you know what's happened, I don't think we've got enough butter to make the cakes?' Emma speaking with emphasis, hand on hip, head to one side.

'I think the shop round the corner might be open. Shall I go and buy some?'

'But have you got any money?' Emma would muse.

'I'm not sure if I've got enough. What are we going to do?'

On another occasion in the park she took us through a low hedge-tunnel in a follow-the-leader game, me crawling on hands and knees behind her.

Emerging cramped and dishevelled at the other end, Emma was nowhere in sight. Instead, a pair of classic, thick-wedged, black shoes with, as I slowly straightened up brushing twigs from my hair, a police officer atop.

'I was following a child,' I said, sounding at my least convincing.

'I promise.'

In the house, Emma showed more than a passing interest in the piano which stood in the corner of the living room by the French windows. A good position to play from, the garden and length of the room both in view from the piano stool.

Visiting children had sometimes gravitated towards it, and quickly lost interest, but Emma was drawn to the instrument. It continued to attract her.

Initially I suggested she should sing along to the music I played.

'I can't,' she said, emphatically shaking her head. 'I don't know how to sing.'

When I said everybody could sing if they wanted, she twisted away from me, head down – and then:

'I like it when you do it.'

But she still hovered near-by, and I asked her one day to come and press her finger on a key to hear what the sound was like.

This she did willingly, and more and more often. It is a picture I have of her: head to one side, catching the note straight in her ear. Always serious.

It became a pleasure, teaching her simple children's melodies, and hearing these from where I moved round the house – with the occasional call for help when she forgot the next note. She was remarkably quick in picking things up: music as well as words.

Our days were enjoyable and sometimes hard. Her moods went full circle from wonderfully bright to: 'I don't feel well' feet-dragging despondancy. We would be skipping along one moment and soon after she would say she could go no further. And that was it.

A sudden drop in energy dogged Emma. From this young in her childhood I would see vitality drain out of her and spread like a stain on the ground.

On walks to the park near-by we had to stop many a time because her legs would not carry her. She would not dance either, at least not initally. Said that, along with singing, she couldn't do that.

Her bed-times, therefore, were sometimes a relief, me tired from a day of stories, swing-pushing and cajoling too. On occasion, long after she had gone upstairs, I would walk to the top of the house where she slept and watch her, arm thrown back, face peaceful, comfort blanket near-by.

Standing in the dark for a few minutes, looking out over the garden and back to where she lay, I would regret my occasional impatience with her, kiss the top of her head.

Once downstairs I would turn to my last duty of the day. From when she was small, and all the time she stayed with me, her colouring and cutting-out book, pencils and scissors were laid out on the table last thing at night, and a glass of milk with two biscuits put beside them. All this arranged, I would turn off the light.

# Chapter Five

❧

# WHO AM I?

Treatment at the Unit where Emma is staying works on the premise that getting a person with anorexia to eat is not, in itself, enough.

Since the illness is described as 'multi-causal', its treatment is worked out along the same lines, approaching the condition on many different fronts.

So, as well as doctors, nurses and dieticians who work out a food programme and a target weight for each individual, there are many therapies — group and family therapy, art and music — within the Unit's recovery programme.

Plans for her progress through this recovery programme have set off alarm bells in Emma when I next visit. She is like a caged animal, sick, cowed, sweating with fear but also, in some sense, dangerous. Ready to pounce.

She had been told she should have full food — three

meals a day – plus food supplements from now on, and is expected to gain one to three pounds a week.

'I can't do it,' she tells me. 'It makes me feel panicky. I won't be able to manage. It's too much.'

Her voice low, almost inaudible sometimes, she says there is a raging battle inside her between life and death. Living frightens her more than dying.

'Why?' I ask gently.

'I'm petrified,' she cries. 'Everything about life, and about the world, frightens me and I want to go back inside myself and never come out again.'

Eloquently she tells me how unprepared she is to live her life. How she doesn't know anything, how to be in the world, have a job, how to speak to strangers. And how all of this makes her want to retreat, stay in the cocoon of her anorexia.

Sobbing by this time, she says her illness is what she knows. It is her safe place, her life. And the world outside, the one where other people live, is too big and frightening for her.

'I would do anything not to have to face it,' she says. 'Anything is better than that.'

Cradling her, I, too, am almost overwhelmed. A girl with eight GCSEs, who is, as it has turned out, a natural pianist, artist, guitar player, with a lovely singing voice, a quick wit, funny sense of humour and tremendous power of articulation, cannot live because life is too big for her.

I fear, too, the effect of her illness on me: the size and

weight of it and its demands on my life. I have wanted to be the 'extra' for Emma, the special person, like a favourite aunt, who will give her treats, cheer her up, be there for her to turn to.

She has become important to me, but my life is full of friends, relatives, travel, work and it's hard to find time to give more.

Emma records this time in her diary:

*I came so very close today to refusing the food i was given – so so close, and it felt like a raging battle was (and is) going on inside me and i wish i could just give in and return to my black and white coffin . . .*

*my body has tightened up, my breathing has quickened and i'm feeling tense and nervous, as though my whole self is anticipating 'something'. It's like this now, when i've eaten, or, as it usually feels, when i've given in . . .*

*That path [relapsing] leads to playing an insane game with my own life, risking it to escape the pressures of living. And whilst death's breath sent many a chill down my protruding spine, it also brought with it the soothing whisper of familiarity.*

In her struggle with the forces of life and death inside her, it is clear I am on the side of life. Although I say nothing to try and force Emma to live, and conceal much of my despair at the thought she might not, it is easy to see which way I am pointing.

And, within weeks of visiting her, Emma sets about trying to reduce my possible influence over her and my capacity to help. I find myself under a kind of veiled, but sustained, attack.

She welcomes me on the one hand and denies me on the other: allows me in; locks me out. Will smile at me as I enter the room or, another time, glance disparagingly over her shoulder, as if to say: 'Oh, not you again.'

This is galling. Emma and I have travelled a long way over many years. I would not demean her, she knows that, and I am angry she should do it to me.

Trying to hold my ground, I marvel at how powerfully articulate she is, and I wince, too, at how capable she is of being scornful.

It was me, after all, who made her 'a word child', who taught her to love language and to play with it, to be skilful in using words, rolling sentences round her tongue, revelling in expressing herself.

We invented many a word game as we walked along, deliberately using long words sometimes, fitting them into sentences, waving our arms, gesticulating, enjoying ourselves. Now, I do not in the least bit enjoy being on the receiving end of Emma's attempts to cut me down to size.

On the Unit this takes an unusual course, which I discover one day when a nurse, used to seeing me around, comments about my age.

'We thought you'd be about eighteen,' she says, smil-ingly. 'Emma described you as her friend and we were expecting someone her own age.'

On the face of it, just a pleasant comment, but, as I swiftly discover, a subtle piece of sabotage from Emma. For she has said nothing more about me to the staff on the Unit. Nothing at all.

She hasn't talked about my caring for her as a child, the fact that I have known her almost all her life. She has concealed the whole lot.

And it explains the odd feeling I have, attending her first case meeting – doctors, nurses, psychotherapists, dieticians all present – that they haven't a clue who or *what* I am. They look surprised when I speak as someone who has known Emma for a long time and whom she confides in.

These meetings, where Emma is present, are important. They assess how she is, how she is responding to treat-ment, and, eventually, make plans for her 'release'.

When she is asked, at this first meeting, how *she* sees things, she says practically nothing, as if she has no voice. Yet we agreed, before we went in, about things she was going to say concerning her individual psychotherapy. She is not responding to it, is subverting this avenue of help too – but a part of her knows she is doing this and is terri-fied of having it withdrawn.

'Tell them,' I say, as we wait to go in. 'They're here to help you.'

Yet she stays silent and, when it looks as if the moment will pass, I say it for her.

It will be a few years after events like these, when I have an overview of Emma's illness, that I will be able to accept, or believe fully, the battle she is involved in between seeking help and rejecting it.

Emma has, as she describes it, 'two sides that fight' inside of her: the white knight; and the destroyer.
She uses the colours white and black for life and death, for purity and oblivion.

Colours are important to her and she writes of life as rainbow-coloured, life not as it is now, but as it might be: dancing, singing, enjoying music, moving freely. At this time, though, there are only the two colours of her pitched sides; frightened Baby Emma and her destructive older sister.

*please please don't, i promise i'll do anything you want, just don't make me have a heart attack.*

*Shut up. I don't care about your stupid baby feelings. Just pull yourself together and grow up . . . you disgust me . . . weeping about 'poor little Emma' . . . stop indulging yourself . . . you know you can fool anyone, and then when we get home I'll cut you and rip you . . . and that's how we live, that's our way. i hurt <u>you</u> – <u>you</u> let <u>me</u>. Fair . . .*

*I want to kill you.*

Who wins when the opponents seem so equally

matched? The struggle is palpable and is what I see in Emma: a battleground. A terrible sight, for Emma is twice torn and many times wounded, switching as she does from side to side, giving and receiving the wounds she inflicts.

Yet the Emma I know understands the difference between good and bad, which is what I hold on to, that somehow she will come to want to console her young, frightened self.

But, then, her breathlessness, the change in her voice as it breaks when she speaks, crying, sobbing, shouting that she is worthless, 'a lump of shit' and does not deserve my help.

Her pain so visible, her courage, too, she is wrung out, torn, trying, chasing inside of herself for somewhere to be at peace — for a safe place.

For me, in all this, there is a continuing kaleidoscope of emotions, from a wish to move towards her, to the need for distance from this sick person.

Emma's deathliness makes me want to retreat and, as they become apparent, so do her lies. At war as she is within herself, I cannot be sure of the level and extent of her self-deception and whether her lies are a defence against me helping too much too soon, or an attack or, indeed, both at the same time. Does she even know she speaks them? Sometimes they seem deliberate, but at others, not.

I am brought low at times with other struggles: to try and separate the girl I knew from this treacherous illness;

to work out which bits of her are which: which is Emma; which is anorexia.

There is one safe wordless place, however. When I hold Emma for the hug which she does not ask for, but never says no to, she is not at war.

Leaning on me, she yields, and stays like that, still and quiet, for a long time. As with the child I came to know, there is something about being held close which keeps the bogeyman away, staves off her demons, makes her world safe.

# Chapter Six

≈

## OLDER THAN HER YEARS

Arriving at my house as a six-year-old, Emma would wriggle out of her knapsack in the hallway, dropping it off her back onto the floor. Free of it, she would clump upstairs to her room. Impatient to get there, she would push on up the next flight of stairs at speed, feet thumping on the stair carpet as she went.

The first few minutes were like this. Her checking the territory, looking around, clocking things. Then, inspection over, back downstairs and music.

I had made inroads into Emma's 'I can't do that' defences by this time and we often began her visit with a song or two at the piano or a dance to one of our favourite records.

A tape of us both at this time, made one Friday night after tea, plays back Emma's voice, clear and tuneful as she stands next to me at the piano. The same voice is loud, boisterous, as we produce an impromptu sketch.

But what Emma brought with her on these visits

troubled me, beginning with her cloth bag, her knapsack, which smelled of smoke, as did everything in it.

Colleen was a heavy smoker, their flat small, and besides the smell on Emma's socks, underwear, spare jumper, there was their drabness. No white vest, nothing pretty. Everything grey, as if all washed together.

Taking the clothes out, I would find a hanger, or drape them over the back of a chair to try and air the smell out of them. But it clung.

Her belongings seemed to reflect not just the lack of money at home, with her mother struggling to provide for them both, but Colleen's subdued spirits. She seemed to have little energy for her daughter.

Although vivacious sometimes in adult company and, indeed, with other children, Colleen is low, flat, with Emma. Formal, almost, in the way she speaks to her, it is as if Emma is someone only to be organised, like a job, rather than a girl to be enjoyed and loved.

This made Emma cautious, hemmed in, unpractised, as I learned many years later. Her early attempts at dancing were, indeed, awkward. She looked like someone placing or putting her arms and legs somewhere, rather than allowing them to move or respond to the music.

There was also her heaviness. Not her sturdy weight, but how she moved. She took smaller steps than she needed to as if afraid to stride out. Yet, as she grew in self-esteem, she had many talents locked up inside her and much to express.

Coming across my guitar one day, she picked out a tune on it, just like that. Soon she would sing a song whenever you asked and dancing was a must in her weekends.

Emma's initial physical awkwardness mirrored her mother's. Colleen held herself badly, shoulders hunched and heavy, as if weighed down. Yet she was pretty, with fair hair, Emma's large eyes, and a lovely warm smile.

But this prettiness was hidden most of the time, kept under wraps. Colleen seemed to show only her plain face to her daughter and Emma reflected this back and out, into the world of her relationships with other people where you did not see how lovely she was at first glance.

Neither were Emma's American relations in evidence in these early years. No one visited from the States and Colleen seldom spoke of her brothers and sisters, five of them, nor of her own parents.

The relationship between Emma and her mother, difficult from when I first knew them, did not improve. They stood back from each other, or at least Colleen did from Emma.

At one of Emma's birthday parties – her fifth, I think – Colleen sparkled with other children, but not with her daughter.

I tried to make up for it, by treating the Birthday Girl as special, but Emma sensed what was happening and a number of times, face troubled, she looked towards where her mother sat, at the kitchen table, with another child on her lap. Once or twice Emma went over to try and establish her place as the child her mother liked best. But holding back, not knowing what to say, body twisting awkwardly, she failed and the other child stayed central.

For her part, Colleen continued to be dutiful with her daughter in a hard-pressed sort of way. She had the demands of a full-time job and, when she came home at night, the needs of a small child. Smoking was her escape. A smoke-cloud hung between them both and when Emma, as a younger child, tried to cross through it, she was fended off.

With Colleen sitting in her usual place at the kitchen table, cigarette in the ashtray, head bent over a crossword, Emma would sometimes accidentally knock the cigarette off its perch trying to grab her mother's attention.

Sometimes the cigarette was in Colleen's hand, and Emma would be told to look out, keep away, watch what she was doing. In those days, at home, Colleen was seldom without a cigarette. A sign of how hard she was finding life.

For Emma, her mother's smoking was a barrier and she formed an intense dislike of it.

'I hate cigarettes,' she would say, stamping hard on the ground on one of our walks. 'I wish my mother didn't smoke.'

As the relationship between Emma and her mother became increasingly distant, I trod a difficult line between protecting Emma and supporting Colleen who was Emma's provider and chief protector and who needed to be strong for both of them.

I hoped that by having Emma visit me, Colleen would get the breaks she needed, time to rest and, also, to go out and enjoy herself.

Colleen, in turn, always welcomed the time I spent with Emma, showing no resentment at the way her daughter was bright and amenable with me and not with her: 'It's nice to know she's good with someone,' would be Colleen's response to my saying Emma had been no trouble.

When Emma was six, Colleen and I took her on a holiday to Devon to stay with friends of mine who were sharing a large country house.

The photographs I took of Emma and Colleen that holiday show two people sitting on a low wall, side by side, shoulders touching, but nothing else: both looking at the camera but no sign they are together.

On this trip, what was already obvious became more so. Emma was not at her best with Colleen and vice versa. With Emma, in the car, or on a walk, Colleen's voice was weary or admonishing. And, for her part, Emma was sulky and difficult to be with.

On holiday a year later, in Wales this time, matters were worse, an August week where it rained, solidly, implacably, all the while we were there.

Staying with members of my large family: my mother, aunt and a motley array of cousins all squashed into a weather-battered old caravan on the Gower Coast, the cramped conditions did not help.

On the second day, walking on the beach in the downpour,

no sign of respite, Emma said, plaintively, how much she had wanted to swim in the sea: 'I was looking forward to it.'

'OK,' I said. 'In we go. It'll be warmer in there than it is out here.'

The tide fully up, or so I thought, there was little distance to walk, so the three of us – Colleen too – stripped to our underwear and in we raced.

The sea *was* warmer, and we had a high old time in the waves, water beneath, rain above, heads bobbing, lots of splashes, shouts and laughter.

We stayed quite a while and then, as we swam to shore, there, heading to greet us, strung out in an ever-widening line, were our belongings, like flotsam, bobbing through the waves.

'Look, the sea's bringing our clothes to us,' giggled Emma.

'Oh blast,' says me. 'Now we're in trouble.'

Spurred on by the thought of a long walk back to the caravan without them, Colleen and I set to. A tee-shirt heading for Ilfracombe, an anorak stopped on its way to Land's End, we dived and scooped again and again, bringing them in to Emma as she played 'clothes monitor' on the beach.

A sock was all we lost, probably halfway to France by this time.

Still shouting and giggling as we struggled into our sea-sodden clothes, we could not wait to get back to the others – to boast of our adventure.

This was the only time I remember seeing Emma and

Colleen positively happy in each other's company, both of them relaxed, calling to each other through the waves.

But back in the confines of the caravan, Emma and Colleen were soon awkward and distant again. And, as the week wore on, more and more so.

By the end of it, my mother had taken me aside: 'What's going on?' she asked. 'She doesn't seem to want the child.'

It was not that simple, though. I do not believe Colleen would have parted with her daughter. But there was something in her, some deep constraint, which stopped her giving Emma what she gave others – affection, spontaneity, liveliness, and the love which Emma yearned for. Free of restraint, for an hour, lulled by the sea, she and Emma had played and then returned to being distant.

In my turn, I waited a long time for Emma to show me affection. Aside from the times when I first knew her when she put her arms up to be carried, she was physically undemonstrative. Staying that way for many years, she expressed herself through words, smiles, shrugs, gesticulations, but not through touch.

Even holding hands was for crossing roads, or some practical reason, like a game, and not for fondness. She seemed unaware of physical contact. And, seemed, also, to manage without it.

And, in a sense, Emma seemed robust. She went about her business in the world as if it were that – business. She addressed herself to matters in hand, applied herself to simple tasks, to doing things, in her own serious, child's way. Much as her mother did, in her world of adult duties.

As she got older, Emma was not backward in asking for what she wanted and sticking to her guns, as with the telly – the place she continued to go back to. However many fun things I filled Emma's days with, it remained her default position for many years.

In the end, though, with me refusing to watch with her most of the time, she would come and find me where I might be reading, writing a letter, or cooking. 'Can we do something now?' she would ask.

Seeing Emma on a regular basis, I had had to accept, long since, her need of me. I was, indeed, a substitute 'aunt' and more.

The 'more' concerned me, for in the demands and pleasures of a full life, I struggled sometimes to find enough time for her visits. But in five years of knowing her, Emma had, indeed, got me to 'lift her up' and I did not feel I could walk away.

As time went on, Emma's pleasure in her stays with me produced another problem. She looked forward to her visits to my place with gusto and determination and began to be more and more distressed when she had to leave.

It began with 'when can I come again?' and escalated, by the time she was seven to: 'I want to come and live with you. Why can't I come and stay here?'

The usual way for her to try and stay on was to say she had a tummy ache, had to lie down, could not walk home or get in the car.

These occasions were distressing and when I took her back our partings were miserable and I regretted, too, leaving Colleen with a despondent child.

I felt helpless, but then what did I expect I asked myself. Colleen and Emma were poor company for each other and this seemed unalterable, at least for now.

Which is how I came to indulge a fantasy. As Emma grew older, things would get better, I said to myself. They do. Time would change things. Children grow up, learn to cope, emerge from painful pasts with surprising tenacity and cheerfulness.

Thus armed, I set, unconsciously, about the task of doing damage of my own, speeding Emma on through childhood, mainly through talking to her and educating her lively, inquisitive mind. As if being able to reason, in itself, would save her.

Willing her to grow fast, it was something she would never recover from – being older than her years.

# Chapter Seven

ↄঙ

## SMOKE-SCREENS OF HER OWN

Seeing her on the Unit, I am unaware of Emma's copious record-keeping. Between the ages of seventeen and nineteen, she has written half a dozen diaries.
And there are many before that.

Emma's determination to have her illness is described graphically in these many journals, as is a frequent change of heart, and her wish both to perpetuate what she is doing and to choose not to die.

Her diary entries are like her weight, up and down, round and round, full of repeated resolve and, also, of ambivalence. Signposts pointing both ways at the same time.
Just before being admitted to hospital in 1998 she writes:

*i don't want to live but I haven't yet chosen death, and until i make up my choice i'm having neither one forced upon me . . .*

*i want this act of self-destruction to be recorded, documented, so that i never forget i did it. anorexia is a fog in my memory, my descent into madness . . .*

*if ever i want to revisit this hell i'm currently in, it will be there for me to know. and i can read my words, my history, my life and know that i've done all this already, and it would be so, so pointless to redo what's already been done . . .*

*Life has so much more to offer than this non-life . . .*

*But first I want to get worse. i once weighed about 5 stones 10 lb. i want to get there again . . .*

*i want to experience it as i now am – with me at the controls, hurtling this body into oblivion . . .*

*As my weight drops, as my silence and refusal of help grows, as my cuts multiply and i drop deeper into this filthy underworld of hurt, i can feel a strength burning in me, flaring up when people try to care, try to oppose my goal of the ultimate agony.*

The Emma I know, then and now, would cringe over a phrase like 'the ultimate agony' used to describe her own state, but she is struggling with extremes, unable to control what she is doing:

*i hate myself so much, so passionately, but i'm too weak to do anything about it . . .*

*Part of me is getting such immense pleasure from my physical deterioration . . . Thinner and thinner and with each bone that rises to the surface of my shrinking form i will be one step closer . . . to the point . . . where i've harnessed death and chosen life . . .*

*i want to be flinging myself full force against brick walls, jumping in front of traffic, breaking bones, and i despise myself for being too gutless to do it.*

It is a popular thought that writing things down acts as a catharsis and moves you forward. It can do the opposite, be a form of escapism, a substitute for life, for living, and hold you back as you go round and round the same track.

So much of the writing in Emma's diaries is like a lava flow and she like an active volcano, insensible to the outpourings which flood out of her. Unexamined by a mind outside her own, by someone whom she will allow to stem the flow, the words just keep on coming.

And, in the end, it is her body, or a realisation of something physical, which is the prompt to life-saving action.

*i feel very clever because i'm vomiting a lot . . . but am taking my potassium whenever there's an interval between binges and so it balances out.*

*i feel clever that i can lose weight without having to worry about my heart stopping.*

Emma agrees to go into hospital soon after, because:

*[although] i don't want to get better yet, i think that getting worse outside of hospital is going to kill me . . .*

*This is like being drained of life. There's a force in my stomach, my chest, a great suction which is causing me to cave in on myself . . . Tightness in my chest, i'm all too aware of my heart, and its exact position within my ribcage . . .*

*it feels like the force of gravity is pulling at me, pulling down down down. It's getting harder to fight it. like my body is somehow transforming itself into lead. My body is eating itself. A good square meal of muscle and organ tissue. i can't even taste the life i'm eating.*

Within a few days of this entry, on Sunday 19 April 1998, Emma is brought into the Unit to be taken care of. The thing she does, and does not, want.

But, although she keeps these entries to herself, she has let me in at last. This is the first time I have seen her regularly since childhood, been on the inside of her illness, and I know I must hang on.

I know, too, that I am the 'scold' in Emma's life at this time, the figure who stands for boundaries which she needs and both does and does not want – yet has asked for.

I find my new role painful. For, in Emma's childhood, I was the fun in her life, the person she came to for dancing, singing, laughter and respite. But, in the face of her illness, I cannot have what *I* would wish for, Emma as a nineteen-year-old healthy young woman.

In the next few weeks Emma is at her most needy and I *believe* her battle. I can see it in her, see her being pulled apart from the inside: backwards; forwards; life; death; resolve; despair. Hope. Terror.

Seeing how terrified she is, it is easy to offer comfort, to spend much of my time cradling her as she talks in a low, frightened voice: anxious; questioning too.

'How is life beautiful?' she asks one evening, from her usual position, draped over me on the bed. 'Tell me, again.'

They have been food for her over the years, these stories, some from my own childhood, of adventures and travels in beautiful places: swimming with dolphins, and among multi-coloured fish; walking over the mountains in Crete; watching a family of rhino cross an African plain; and, one of her favourites, the young elephant who arrived one afternoon to play with my brother and me in a Tanzanian garden.

She continues to ask for these over and over, has listened attentively to their retelling: 'tell me about the elephant again', 'describe the fish'.

'Can we go to Crete if I get better?' she asks on one of my visits. 'And to Africa?'

'Yes,' I say. 'But you would have to be fit to climb those hills and survive in the bush.'

A small turning point happens around this time, something which eases the battle a little. At least, I think so.

Holding her one evening, she limp and sweating, terrified, again, of living, and crying out: 'I can't, I can't. It's too difficult,' it suddenly seems to me that it *is*.

Why should I, why should anyone, expect her to go on fighting in this way, torn apart, minute by minute? Although I want her to live, I do not believe I have the right to impose it on her, to demand it.

Struggling to find a response to her cries for help, one which does not deny her pain or collude with it, I say no one who cares about her would ask her to do what is too difficult.

'I'll love you whether you live or die.'

Going home that night, I have anguish of my own. Will she use these words as permission to give up? Will letting her know she is loved, help to kill her?

And, if this were to happen, how would I live with that?

# Chapter Eight

~&

# A Hot Day in the Park

Emma's signals of distress were present in her poor eating from a young age. For all her time with me as a child, food was a trial for her.

On a weekend, she might have a boiled egg for tea, with half the soldiers left uneaten. She would eat a biscuit and milk later on, a tiny amount of cereal and a small piece of an apple for breakfast, a sandwich and drink for lunch, and so on. Salad was not acceptable to Emma. Neither were most vegetables.

Cheese on toast was OK, and so was toast and honey, but Emma ate only just enough to keep going and never a full, proper meal. Painting book, games, cards, all of these were fine spread out on the table. But not cooked food.

Trying to involve her in meal-times, she would happily lay the table, knives and forks in the right places, and bake cakes with me as well. But as soon as the real stuff arrived, a cooked main course, and we sat down to the business of eating, Emma was cagey. Her body twisted away, she was reticent, oblique. Eyes sliding from my gaze, there was something evasive about her which did not respond to anything I said, or did.

Sensing the size of the problem, in her early days with me, when she was four, five, I bought pretty plates and made sure food was presented nicely: cut up in small pieces to tempt her.

I thought it would produce results, that Emma's difficulty with food was one of being given time, of feeling cared for while she ate. It worked a little, in that I could see something in her yield as I coaxed her like this – but not very much, nor for long.

By the age of eight, Emma would watch cheerfully, chatting away, as I enjoyed a proper meal, but she did not want it for herself. Something small on toast: beans, an egg, was what she had instead. The fish and chips we had together sometimes, she seemed to like, but did not eat much of.

When I tried to *make* her eat what I had cooked by refusing to prepare something different, she ate nothing, went hungry and was listless, miserable – afraid? I was, after all, someone she liked and trusted. Would I turn against her? Would food come between us?

Speaking to Colleen about it, her weariness was obvious, and I had seen the extent of the problem while visiting them:

Colleen calling Emma away from the TV for a meal; Emma coming in and saying she didn't want it. Colleen hoped she would grow out of it.

An incident in the park at this time was troubling too. Staying with me one summer's night, while Colleen was away, I had picked Emma up on foot and we were going back to my place via the children's paddling pool.

It was very hot and Emma, in her strapless sundress, fair skin exposed, was a target, I feared, for the burning sun.

By the pool, discovering there was no sunscreen in Emma's knapsack, and afraid she might burn, I said she could have just ten minutes in the water, and we could come back again tomorrow. Pulling her sundress over her head, swimsuit underneath, Emma looked even more vulnerable and I waited anxiously.

Ten minutes later, the trouble began. No, she wasn't coming out of the pool into the shade.

Reasoning with her, I explained again: no sunscreen; hot sun; her fair skin. She might get nasty things like blisters. And we wouldn't want that would we?

Or did she?

I had occasionally seen a mother do it, drag a wailing child along behind her in the park, and had thought: 'Why doesn't she stop and talk to the child?'

And, here I was, dragging Emma towards a large chestnut tree and some shelter.

All the way back to my place it went on, a bit of dragging, a few toppling steps, me stopping now and then to see if I could find out what was ailing her.
Shaking her head, saying nothing, she continued to resist me.

But, at last, the safety of the house, with the welcome shade and cool of the basement hallway and a breeze through the windows. She was out of harm's way.

Walking through to the kitchen to calm myself, a sudden wail sounded from the living room. Rushing through, there was Emma, under the piano, where she had flung herself down to sob over and over again: 'You don't love me.'

Telling her that of course I did, and why would she think I didn't, Emma remained silent when I asked, gently, what had made her so upset. It was the first time, however, she let me hold her, both of us leaning against the piano a while, me shushing her sobs, stroking her hair.

Looking back on this incident, Emma had picked up on something, I believe, and was reacting to it. It was the first time Colleen had stayed out when Emma came to me, and there was something else. Colleen was with Paul, a man she had recently met and would marry the following year.

Emma knew instinctively there was a change in her mother's life and one which might threaten their already fragile relationship.

During this summer, Emma began to sit curled up with me as we spent companionable times together on the settee, chatting, listening to music, reading, me telling her increasingly sophisticated stories.

Sometimes, head on my lap, she would ask for the story of how we met in the pub.

'Will you write it in a book?' she asked me, and I said that, yes, one day, I would.

She often did this, asked for familiar stories, ones of when she was small: 'tell me about when I first came to stay with you' and 'tell me, again, about the policeman and you in the tunnel'.

Most children do this, ask for stories to be repeated, but the stories were more than reassuring for Emma. They were urgent, food to make up for her emotional hunger, the absence of relations and a family history.

The incident in the park notwithstanding, Emma's walking had improved, and we had fun exploring London. A family of stone rhinoceroses were part of the city's system of moveable sculptures at the time. In a small green area on the South Bank, I have pictures of her sliding down their backs, arms wide open, laughing.

Strolling along together, we fed geese, squirrels and, from the banks of a local canal, listened in amazement, one day, to a whistling duck. There it was. We could see its beak opening, and then this whistle.

Silly me, it was a wigeon, of course.

As Emma came into her ninth year, growing up fast,

she was intelligent, quick, affectionate and, with me, obliging.

There was the evening I went out to get fish and chips for us both, as a treat. Emma staying at home in the warm, where she preferred to be at the end of a school day, I said I would be no more than ten minutes. She knew, in any case, not to open the door to anyone.

Back a short while later, I was met by a cleared-up living room: newspapers in a pile; piano music too; guitar upright against the wall.

'I've cleared upstairs in your study as well,' said Emma, proudly.

'Oh,' I said, trying to conceal the despair in my voice.

Some writers have photographic memories for shapes and where sentences are on separate, scattered pages. Here the pages were, in a squared-off pile. Unrecognisable. Dead. I gulped.

'Oh,' I said again. 'Haven't you been busy, you've done a marvellous job. Thank you.'

Later over the meal, I ventured: 'Emma, if you decide to tidy up again, please would you leave the study *un*tidy.'

She gave me one of her long looks.

'You see,' I said, 'some writers work better that way.'

'Do *you*?' she asked, straight to the point.

'Oh, I vary,' I said airily, not wanting to hurt her feelings.

Around this time, 'Alfred' came to stay. King Alfred, as she called Alan, a flat-mate who stayed for around eighteen months to help pay the mortgage.

The house large enough for him to have his own living room, we shared bathroom, kitchen and Emma.

Divorced with children of his own, Alan enjoyed her company and she his. They were soon involved in boisterous games, dashing up and down stairways, hiding, calling, giggling.

Princess Emma and King Alfred were a feature for a while and I was glad Emma, who was unfriendly to men and ignored them in the main, liked Alan so much. Sometimes, going on outings together, he bought her ice-creams and indulged her, like a good father might.

After one such day out, I prepared a special meal, a long time in the kitchen producing something tasty which Emma, as usual, refused to eat.

Angered, I was blunt: 'Either you eat it or I don't cook anything special again.'

Distressed, blushing, squirming slightly, Emma said, genuinely I believe, that she could not eat it, did not know why, but 'just couldn't'.

We left it there.

And Emma was sturdy, not thin. Knowing people have different metabolic rates, I thought perhaps she burned calories slowly and felt there was nothing more I could do. Either she and I were going to fight over her poor eating or I would get on with providing other food: stories, music, fun, affection.

The answer to the riddle of how Emma stayed sturdy without eating very much did not lie in metabolic rates, though. As her hospital records show, from this age and, in a less deliberate way, from when she was younger, Emma was set on a path, her way with food and starvation already begun.

# Chapter Nine

❦

## EMMA IN LIMBO

The struggle in Emma is fierce, palpable, as I visit her at the Unit, but she is eating and her weight is rising, past six and a half stone, heading towards seven.

The battle in her between the size and unpredictable nature of 'life' and a fixed, controllable 'coffin place' where she fantasises about death continues:

> . . . life is bloody terrifying. Things happen unexpectedly and without warning . . .
> Life scares me. And when i'm scared i reach out for something safe – anorexia; bulimia.

Emma separates anorexia and bulimia in her diaries. For some experts they are the same, phases of what is called anorexia nervosa.

Many cases of anorexia involve a combination of bulimia

– of bingeing followed by enforced vomiting – followed, eventually, by starvation.

Bulimia by itself and 'restricting anorexia' (starvation which does *not* involve binge/purging) are both less common as individual illnesses.

So, it is not unusual for people suffering from anorexia to go through the kind of loops Emma did; starving, then over-eating, then vomiting again.

And, as her weight rises by a kilo or more a week, Emma, on the upward curve of the loop, is volatile.

> i notice my body growing. the bulge of my stom-ach; the flapping of flesh on my thighs, the puff-ing out of my cheeks . . . it's not a pleasant feeling.

But, on the same day she also writes:

> music/singing/dancing and laughing with people, read-ing, moving – all that is very much alive . . . it (the feeling that comes from gaining weight) *doesn't* seem like much to sacrifice.

Then, back into ambivalence, duality, threat. After 'sacri-fice' she writes the ominous words 'not yet', followed by:

> And i do need to be a healthy weight <u>anyway</u>.

The 'anyway' is Emma hedging her bets, for to starve yourself successfully, systematically, you need to begin with weight to lose.

> *I need to get back to a reasonable state of health so I can enjoy my bulimia again.*

Around this time, plans are being made for Emma to leave the Unit. She will remain a day-patient, attending for music, art, group and individual therapy, but a shortage of beds means hers is needed at the end of an eight-week stay.

She will have to go.

Where to?

Between one of my visits and the next, the problem becomes urgent because Emma has decided not to return to her mother's home:

> *The part of me that wants to return home to live is the part of me that wants to cling to my eating disorder . . .*
>
> *That's the part that can't ever relax, that's desperately unhappy. The part of me that's reluctant to take risks, face fears, grow up and face life.*

Emma tells me she wouldn't be able to live at home without being bulimic, that home means either over-eating or under-eating.

'It feels like something that can't be repaired.'

Her alternative is alarming. She says she is going to stop a few days or a week with one friend and then another, sleeping on floors if necessary, until the hospital, as it is trying to do, finds her accommodation.

But most of the friends she tells me about are, themselves, in various stages of anorexia. Although living in the outside world, part recovered, they are not strong, I imagine, nor wise enough to give Emma the structure and boundaries she needs.

A case meeting in a few days' time will result in her being officially discharged as an in-patient and I fear for Emma. She is not ready to leave.

Before this meeting, we struggle, she and I. Emma is fragile, vulnerable, on the one hand and, on the other, imperious and demanding.

And I have problems of my own.

I have begun a three-year training course to be an Alexander Technique teacher, have taken on work for a writers' union – and am writing, seeing friends, going out as usual. It is a bad time to be asked to give more.

Yet, as in the past, abandoning Emma is not an option. Friends and family I talk to about it know, as well as I do, there are only two alternatives. Either I stand by her, or Emma sleeps on friends' floors, unable to cope, drifting back into danger. The 'or' is not an attractive prospect.

In this period Emma is at her most needy and dismissive. In her needy guise, she wants to be helped and in her other 'I-can-manage' mode she wants her illness in her own way, at her own pace – without my intervention.

For my part, I will not go along with the aspect of Emma's illness which denies me and what I have done for her. I am too stretched to be taken for granted or badly used – and visiting Emma is only a small portion of what is needed of me on her behalf at this time.
There are meetings, phonecalls and the usual bureaucratic frustration.

Like my appointment the previous week with a social worker, Therese, temporarily assigned to Emma's case. A short, stocky woman in her early thirties, with fair hair and a rather officious manner, she wishes to see me to discuss Emma, but insists I travel to her. An hour there. An hour back.

In her office, documents and forms in hand, Therese wants answers to questions that cannot be answered in one or two words.

'What is Emma's relationship with her mother like?'

I hesitate, wondering where to begin.

'Is it good or bad?' Therese asks.

'It's more complicated than that,' I say. 'It's a long story, there were definitely problems from when Emma was young – and a reason for her to be resentful . . .'

I suggest I give Therese an overview of what I saw of Emma's childhood to put her relationship with Colleen in context.

Politely, Therese lets me know she would prefer to get the information she wants her way. She moves on:

'How often does Emma see her father?'

'At what age did her problem with food begin?'

Well, around six, probably, or maybe seven, or maybe, even, before then. Definitely a problem by the age of eight, but not clinically, you might say, until she was fifteen. Which age to pick?

Emma says of Therese soon after: 'She doesn't listen to me. She asks me something and if I don't give her a reply she wants, she doesn't take any notice. It's like she doesn't hear me.

'Sometimes I feel like giving her what she wants, even if it's not true.'

I ask Emma not to do this, tell her to speak the truth because Therese will be writing up what Emma gives her and using it at case meetings.

Better, I say, not to give misleading information.

But my interventions in Emma's life, while asked for, are also deeply resented. As Emma wants her illness her way, so it is with her recovery, and my part in it.

While I am mentioned patchily in Emma's diaries, and in differing lights, there is one long sequence, a short while after this conversation about Therese, where she writes graphically of her wish to kill me, her 'I's' in full capital letters.

*I hate Carol. I really really hate her . . . Right now I want to strangle her, to beat her body to the ground . . . until I'm standing tall above her . . . I, for once victorious.*

Helping someone with anorexia is a battle of wills in which neither person must be broken and where one must be allowed to give way and to slip quietly out of the 'cold hallways' which beckon her. As in all battles, positioning is crucial, as is timing.

I, who was, as Emma later describes it, 'the happy place of her childhood', have information that would help to save her. But she is not ready yet.

# Chapter Ten

✌

# A GIANT APPETITE

As the chosen adult in Emma's life, someone she can confide in, and who will visit and care for her, I am also a substitute target for the resentment and anger she has stored up against her mother.

Emma sees Colleen only once during her stay on the Unit – in her first week – and, as she notes in her diary, was violently ill afterwards.

She decides not to see Colleen again and, a short while later, asks for me instead.

The reason Emma gives me for her distress after the meeting with her mother is that she desperately wanted to hear that Colleen was grieving, sorrowing for her – Emma – being so ill. She wants to hear the words, 'I'm sorry I let you down.'

Instead, Colleen, at her most cautious and restrained, produces something subtly, and distinctly, different. She is, naturally, *sorry* Emma is ill, is what Emma tells me she says. Of course she is. But, no, she is not sorrowing for her daughter's plight. She is upset, as any mother would be, but she goes to work as usual, gets on with her life, as you have to.

She is not brought low. Which is where Emma wants, needs, her to be.

I can see why Colleen cannot – dare not – submit to Emma's will. For Emma is articulate, fierce, grown now, and, I believe, harbours a wish to do to Colleen what she wrote of doing to me.

Unsurprisingly, Colleen is not up for this. Her hope, her fantasy has been Emma 'growing out of it' and Time doing its work. Instead, she is faced, ten years on, with the problem accumulated: a nightmare.

'I know what you want, and why,' I say to Emma, 'It's what everyone wants. A mother who is available, loving, capable, who worries about us as we go through life.

'But most of us have to let go of this, and I don't believe your mother's going to change. I don't think she can afford to.'

There is a part of Emma which understands this, and another which is furious and hurt.

'Why won't she just *feel* for me? Is it such a big deal for her to say she's really sorry and mean it for once?'

As anger gives way to tears, I can do nothing but hold Emma, let her sob.

She feels abandoned and frustrated. The needy part of

her wants Colleen to take notice, and the angry part wants revenge. But Colleen is unavailable for either.

It is dangerous ground for Emma, and she feels she may go under.

> I remember sometimes pushing mum's attention away, because i resented it not being there constantly for me whenever i wanted it, or other times not taking as much as i wanted from her because i didn't want to use up all her love. The times that i pushed her love away was me saying 'you can't love me as much as i need you to, so i'm not having any of your love, and you'll see just how terrible it is for me to be without it . . .'
>
> i badly want to love + care for myself . . . I think that my attitude may have been learnt through my treatment as a child – i always felt like my mum couldn't love me enough for what i needed and she rarely showed me affection except for those times when i was ill or very distressed.

And, later in 1998, after she has begun to respond to therapy:

> EMMA. Sad. Fallen. Drained. Hurting. Child. Woman.

Then, many times over:

*She would have let me die.*

and finally:

*She would have let me die, my mother.*

Without the love she craves Emma is left prey to what she thinks of as the giant, and unassuageable, nature of her appetite – for food and affection:

> *i have a hunger*
> *can never be touched*
> *everything ever*
> *is never enough*

Earlier, in April, before coming back on the Unit she writes:

> *i don't have the guts to face my appetite, for food or for life . . .*
> *If I wasn't such a greedy pig, what I had would be enough; I'm afraid that if I try to lead a normal life, to eat food normally, I will have to face my insatiable appetite – that I can never, in the whole world, get enough.*

Reading through Emma's diaries, the word leaps out at me. *My* word, 'enough', spoken with emphasis around midnight a few months after the incident of dragging Emma through the park.

Her mother is away for a week, and Emma staying at my place from where I take her to school each day and, at night, try to console her. For Colleen is on holiday with Paul, the man she had begun a relationship with some months earlier, with Emma left behind.

I think the timing is appalling. Emma should have been allowed to get to know Paul before he and Colleen went away. Even staying with me, a happy place, she will feel abandoned. But, in the months leading up to meeting Paul, Colleen has been low, sounding more and more burdened. Sensing her desperation, I do not refuse to have Emma and, indeed, where else would she go?

On the first night of her mother being away, aware of Emma's sleeplessness, I go up, around midnight, to where she is sitting up in bed with the light on, pillow propped behind her, twisting the sheet between her clenched hands, trying to break it apart.

'My mummy doesn't love me,' she says vehemently. 'I'd be better off in an orphanage. At least then the person who took me home would want me.'

What can I say? How to acknowledge the reality, the truth of her pain, coupled with the extent of her understanding of it – and at the same time protect her from both? A world without a mother's love? No place for a child.

'It's not that your mother doesn't love you *at all*,' I say, searching for a way through. 'It's that she doesn't love you *enough*. She doesn't love you enough for what you want.'

There it is, the word she repeats over and over in her diaries ten years later, the source of the appetite she feels she cannot conquer.

I think of 'food' phrases and words Emma must have heard as a child many times over, often from me:

'You haven't eaten enough.'

'You must eat more.'

'You won't grow big and strong without eating enough food.'

Listening to me that night, sitting, propped up by pillows, her face serious, Emma's eyes are large with expression. Partly they challenge me:

'Well, now it's as bad as I always knew it would be, what are you going to do about it?'

Partly they are far away, beyond help, distraught.

For the rest of the week, Emma goes to school, comes home, is OK on the surface. But she is heavy with her bag of troubles. Sad. Hurt. Unreachable.

When Emma was young I did what I could to make up for her life at home. I enjoyed her and was glad to have her in my life. Although a child with a great deal of baggage she was bright, cheerful, funny as well, and we were good company for each other.

Trying often to shield Emma from the pain of her poor relationship with her mother, I did not, however, pretend it was otherwise. I believe her world felt grey, difficult,

drab, and my place, a chink of light in it, but rationed.
Not enough.
For how big is enough in a child's world, and what colour
is it?

# Chapter Eleven

❧

## BAD COMPANY

I come to learn many things about anorexia through being Emma's visitor, in particular that people who suffer from it often call the condition their 'friend'. Their illness is what they decide to adopt in the face of unresolvable problems, and is what they have to hold on to. It becomes intrinsic to their identity and, in a sense, understands them.

Anorexics can think of their illness as supporting rather than killing them, and any attempt to take it away as a threat. You might persuade a person to let go of anorexia, but you cannot sever them from it by force. Like many an unsuitable teenage friendship, an adult is relatively power-less to intervene without the risk of making things worse.

I know I must not try and remove Emma's illness from her, or her from her illness. If I try and do that, I will be the enemy who does not understand her as her 'friend' does. I may not even discuss it with her – at least not directly.

Emma may – and does – for along with her continuing involvement with anorexia, she is also ambivalent. She longs to hold on to her friend, but also begins to sense what it does to her.

She writes with revulsion of how low she has been brought:

> The craving [for food] mounts with every mouthful of sweetness . . . I scavenge like a rat for more, and more . . .
>
> I don't want to feed myself, i'm just a messy bit of sordid muck . . .

followed, a few weeks later, by:

> bulimia, my safety net, my security blanket, my friend . . .
>
> I wish i was still hungry so i could eat more. I don't want to say goodbye to the part of me that always craves more . . . who am i without my huge passion for food?

Around this time there are names of foods closely written on the page. At one stage eleven pages of temptingly written edible delicacies, the writing getting smaller and smaller to allow room for more, all beginning with the words:

*Food is filling my mind.*

A few months after this Emma asks herself the question:

*What would happen if i let myself feel the anx-*
*iety without the filter of chaindrinking and over-*
*eating. . . . the undiluted fear? . . .*
*    i've started to run. The race is on. The pace*
*increases with each added piece of information in*
*my head and the momentum of my terror keeps me*
*on the treadmill, preventing me from discovering*
*what waits for me in stillness.*

I believe what awaits Emma, in the place she calls stillness, where anorexia is not, is her battle with her appetite:
for food; for life; for anger; and, possibly, something she
really cannot bear, for revenge.
She has 'lion' dreams a while after this, and writes of 'the
savage beast inside, rampant and wild'.

*i have a lion. His huge body stands tall before me*
*in all its fiery glory, blocking my view of the*
*sun. His deep shadow is cast over me like a thick*
*blanket, and is sometimes comforting, sometimes*
*smothering.*
*    Sometimes i find myself riding on his back . . .*
*and cleansing my filthy, rotting and fermenting*
*insides, when i'm brave enough to snatch a taste of*

*life. But mostly i live in fear of his immense strength.*

*Mostly i just cower in a lonely dirty corner, . . . hiding from the lion i keep locked up inside.*

Locking away appetite, anger, the fullness of life, anorexia helps cover up whatever struggles inside. With its controlling bouts of bingeing and starvation, of trance and half-life, it becomes a shield to fend off despair and longing and what most of us would see as ordinary responsible behaviour.

'Doesn't she care what she does to her family?' people will ask.

'How can she starve herself like that?'
She has fallen into bad company, been influenced from within by something she thought she could control, but which has ended up controlling her.

Experts who have spent years working with anorexia sufferers see the illness as a means of expressing distress – a *symptom*, not a cause. One doctor describes anorexia as a *solution* to an individual's problem, so by treating the solution life is made more difficult.

This would explain why Emma is ruthless in protecting her illness, as if it were her life, rather than the thing which is destroying her.

By June 1998, she is coming up to being twenty, to leaving the Unit as an in-patient and to the most anguished of times. She is being challenged to live, which would mean leaving her 'friend' of five, or maybe fifteen, years behind. How can she think of herself, her life without this?

*I don't have the guts to face my appetite, for food, or for life . . . all i can feel, think, be, right now is worthless, greedy, lazy, selfish, dirty, disgusting pig. me.*

So long as she needs her illness, her solution, Emma fights me and the world to keep it, and I with my armoury of understanding and affection might tip the balance too far too quickly.

To combat my influence, she continues to keep me at bay.

Trying, on one occasion, to bring her round, discussing my place in her life, she treats me as if she is the parent and I a fractious child.

'Why, you're Carol,' she responds condescendingly.

I am not having it:

'We have a history,' I tell her bluntly.

'I'm not just a friend. I'm an adult who's known you almost all your life. You need to accept that.'

I dislike fighting with her, for it is an uneven contest. I can read Emma. I know her. It is difficult for her to hide from me and there is something I have begun to glimpse.

In June 1998, in a period of gaining weight, finding life big, full and often overwhelming, she writes of wanting the rainbow colours of a full spectrum, yet . . . :

*yet still i crave the sight of my own hypnotic gaze
reflecting out at me from the shared mirror of
anorexia and bulimia, numb to life and reality,
existing only in my self-made tortured state.*

I believe Emma's close friendship with her illness, involving the trance-like states which she describes bulimia bringing her, *was* hypnotic and did involve a gaze in a mirror, that of self-identity.

And, in the elaborate defence she constructed to protect her illness, her identity, against threat from outsiders, I think Emma's mirror-friend, her trance, became something she would defend to the death – something to die for.

For this was not a vain glance, the self-absorbed narcissism of 'mirror, mirror on the wall, who is the fairest of us all', but something deathly: a dark, dangerous glass reflecting an altogether different kind of gaze.

*Do you see me? That is me dying. That is me look-
ing in the mirror at my reflection and seeing an
ugly disgusting greedy useless mess, only occasionally glimpsing the reality – a young girl's quest
for a corpse.*

Finding these rare and revealing mirror entries makes me recall that Emma did not like mirrors as a child, at least not ones on the outside.

On the inside it seems she harboured secrets about

herself – bad ones – which I did not know about. That she had been raiding her mother's fridge from the age of eight: refusing to eat what was cooked for her; binge-eating behind Colleen's back.

But she also harbours a wish for another, less oppressive, image in her inner glass. And the one that might counter-balance this 'greedy mess' is the alluring spectre of its opposite: a fragile, food-denying figure, 'a young girl's quest for a corpse'.

*My world is fast becoming dead and emotionless . . . Carol came to visit me today. She's very alive, there's a lot of passion and pain and joy and richness in her life. i envy that . . . i feel so brain dead.*

At the Unit, Emma curled round me, I feel sometimes as if I am holding up a charm or an amulet to ward off her deathliness. My one trump card, something her illness cannot take away, our history and the stories I carry in my head.

'Tell me again . . .' she will say, or 'Do you remember . . . ?' I will ask.

Although anorexia will try, even here, to confound us. Emma's memory is already under attack, and while long-term loss is not common to the illness, Emma suffers both long and short-term gaps. Aware of this, I provide for her, when she will accept it, story-food.

Emma is peaceful in these times, her mirror-friend turned to the wall. Instead Alfred, the wigeon, making tapes together, the day we met and her wish for me to write about it in a book, the hut in the park, clothes floating towards us on the water.

True Stories.

## Chapter Twelve

❧

## THE LOCK-OUT

Around a year after first meeting him, when Emma is nine, Colleen marries Paul.

A dark-haired, softly-spoken draughtsman, he is a great support to Colleen and offers Emma love and support, which she rejects. Not for a long time, more than a decade, will she accept him:

*When Mum married Paul i was resentful . . . i'd see her being affectionate with him, yet she couldn't be with me unless i was ill or distressed . . .*

*Paul was a very positive person there for me, didn't hide his love for me, but i think i must have really resented that the love was coming from him, and not my mum. It seemed like she'd 'got' Paul to do the job of loving me, so she didn't have to.*

Years later, she says:

'I felt my mother gave Paul the job [of loving me]. So he was a substitute.'

Picking her up from school a few months after the wedding for an overnight at my place, Paul is there, too, with some things for her, including sweets. A way, I believe, of letting her know she is not being abandoned.

But she just shouts at him:

'I didn't ask for those kind,' pointing at the sweets. 'I wanted the others.'

Walking away with her I say I would feel angry and upset if she talked to me like that.

I see little of Emma between the ages of ten and fifteen, no more than once every couple of months. Paul having arrived, I think there is less need of the stand-in role I have played in her life. And I do not want to intrude. They are a family now and, after a period of resentment, Emma will surely grow to accept Paul and to enjoy having the father-figure she has missed.

Although part of me is relieved to have more spare time, I miss Emma's stays with me and the closeness we had together.

During this time, Paul and Colleen invite me over for occasional meals. They are both excellent cooks and I look forward to this but, to my surprise, Emma stays mainly shut away in the other room watching TV.

Bothered by this, I remind her she can call me whenever she likes, have a chat, come and stay sometimes, too.

But while pleased to see me, she shows little interest in coming to my place. She seems cut off, isolated, the TV once more her retreat.

The years after Emma leaves primary school are a blur for me. On visits to the flat, I notice how much she is given, and given into, mainly by Paul, with Colleen's tacit, and background, approval.

Her mother withdrawn even further from her, with Paul doing much of the parenting, Emma is increasingly indulged with gifts and sweet things which do not seem to make her happy. She comes to expect, and demand, a great deal, which is not how she used to be.

For me, her bedroom is a nightmare, hundreds of ornaments, toys, cutesy objects, crammed into her small room. They feel oppressive. But she asks for them and is given more and more. None of this seems good for her.

As she approaches eleven her appearance, too, troubles me; she is heavier, seems to do no exercise, develops the same stooped shoulders as her mother and looks as if she doesn't care about herself. And with her friends Emma changes from an intelligent, sensitive person into someone else: loud; uncaring.

She shouts and speaks an aggressive but, for her, awkward, street language.

Having had turbulent teenage years of my own, I accept some of what Emma is doing as a need to test herself, to become independent.

But something is wrong. Emma is not gaining ground, but

losing it, losing herself. For later it becomes clear that by this time, she was secretly longing to die.

Behind her acquisitive exterior, an entry when she is eighteen and looking back at her life gives a desperate picture of what it felt like:

> *Sunday laziness dirty clammy childish delaying and fatness and starving and stuffing in* [food] *and mum and Paul and pocket money and hating hating lonely sad alone ugly terrified shut away unwanted choking barriers shut doors bad TV and homework done last thing and desperation . . .*
>
> *To live your life unseen, unheard and ignored . . . for me it's an enormous hurting hole which in vain i've tried to fill either with food, or the lack of it.*
>
> *But to live your life seen, heard and disregarded . . . i'm terrified of exposing myself as i really am.*

Hiding away and feeling awkward from when she started going to school, Emma had problems with friendships, with feeling different and left out.

Waiting to pick her up from primary school, I noticed her with other children, how she was timid, how she hung back and then pushed herself forward in an obvious, awkward way. For Emma, friendships with children and adults alike were fraught.

*I loved Mary, she was my favourite teacher — i remember once i was really ill, and off school for at least a week . . . it was Mary's birthday and so i sat at home making her loads of cards and pictures and papery things, and put them all into a big envelope i'd made and decorated.*

*I also remember putting in a few Chocolate Eclair sweets, and other bits and pieces . . . I remember feeling unhappy when I went back to school because she never mentioned it. Paul (who had taken the card in) said she'd said Thank You to him (to me), and i remember pestering him for every last detail of her reaction. I know that i wanted to hear that she really loved it, that it was special to her and made her happy (+ like me more).*

Phoning Emma from time to time in her early teens, trying to let her know I was there, but not wishing to interfere, she would have me believe she was enjoying herself being a normal, gregarious teenager. As it turns out, she was spending more and more time binge-eating in her bedroom.

Giggling, she told lies, as she was used to doing by now, about how she was having a terrific time: going out with friends; playing music; having fun.

'So no time for me, then?' I'd ask, half-invitingly.

'When I'm less busy,' would be Emma's cheery reply.

When I asked Paul, or sometimes Colleen, how she really was, the answers were confusing:

Yes, she was going out with friends, from Colleen.

She was spending a lot of time in her bedroom, from Paul. But then, at her age, that was not unusual. Perhaps she was going through a phase.

Emma's fifteenth birthday, and the events which followed, gave a different perspective. The birthday celebration was a meal out. Just the four of us: Emma, Paul, Colleen, me. This is what Emma had asked for, apparently, all of us at dinner together.

Or had something got lost in translation?

For Emma refused to speak to the people she now called her parents. Sitting opposite us in the restaurant, I felt dreadful for them, and for her too. For she must have known how awful this was.

What did it cost her, what was she thinking, feeling, to be this unyielding?

Stuck in the middle, remembering that, in a sense, a version of this had gone on for more than a decade, I was deeply worried where it might lead to. Someone had to call a halt to it. Somehow, Emma had to be challenged, for her own sake.

A few weeks later, on a Sunday afternoon, came the phonecall from Paul. Emma had barricaded herself in her bedroom. She refused to say what was wrong. Would I come over? She might come out for me. Walking to the flat, I dreaded betraying Emma, which is how I felt she would see it.

Paul, who could easily have broken in, did not want to

use force and cause more alarm. My suggestion, to get in professional help with a call to the family doctor was rejected by Colleen. Yet it had gone too far for us, and needed outside assistance. Speaking to Emma through the door, asking, quietly, if she would talk to me, let me in, she remained silent.

Emma would not come out that day, nor did she talk about the incident for many years, but locking herself in followed the news of the death of a young actor, River Phoenix, from a drugs overdose.

It was the shock she needed.

River Phoenix had been Emma's fantasy lover for some time. Kept secretly in the pages of her diary, she 'spoke' to him and, unlike the rest of the world, he 'knew' how she felt. His sudden death gave her something she had longed for – resolve.

Emerging of her own accord two days later, she was withdrawn, ill-looking, altered.

Emma was now on a determined course. The first downward loop of her journey into anorexia had begun.

# Chapter Thirteen

ﻬ

## THE MIRROR INSIDE

As a child, Emma did not accept Paul's place in her life and how much he tried to do for her. In fact, Paul being so extraordinarily patient with her may have made her feel worse about herself.

What she writes most often is how fat, ugly and greedy she is. And, unwittingly, Emma had been indulged, encouraged, in this opinion of herself, for no one had stopped her when she behaved badly. Colleen had not, and Paul's acceptance of her as she was and his unconditional care for her had unwittingly preserved this image.

Desperate for a way to cope with her sense of worthlessness as she entered her teenage years – feeling fat, ugly and frightened of her appetite – Emma secretly hoarded the fake food of a 'love', an infatuation, for the actor, River Phoenix.

*It was during my 'ugly phase' that i cared about River, when i was at secondary school. Because i couldn't take my 'invisible friend' to school with me, i had to leave him at home, so it's no wonder i felt so shitty all day and never ate lunch/any food until i got home and could be with 'him' again. Then i'd have several sandwiches + bowls of cereal + big glasses of juice/chocolate milk + fruits ¢ any snacky things that were around. I think i'd been leaving the love for myself at home all day, and then been coming home to it and trying desperately to make up for the time i was without it, like one big reunion feasting.*

By her fifteenth birthday Emma was already far away from daily life and the reality of our awkward dinner table. Deeply preoccupied with thoughts of River, her fantasy friendship developed into a love affair:

*I'd have little conversations with my imaginary lover, and could sometimes even feel that there was an actual presence there. I'd sit in the armchair in the living room, in the evenings, staying up late watching TV + snacking, imagining that i was sharing the chat . . . Many nights i fell asleep in bed with my arms wrapped around myself, holding in the warm love, not letting any of it escape.*

But it did escape. On Halloween, when he was twenty-three years old, River Phoenix died.

> *I'd convinced myself that my purpose in living was to be with him eventually, and so when he died i felt like someone had ripped out my heart.*
>
> *In seeing myself in so much of River, who i thought was beautiful, i used to manage to give love to myself, so his death was also the death of my love for myself. I stopped eating as soon as i heard the news of his death. I remember my anorexia as being very cold, empty, painful, grey, lonely. I could only love myself if i felt someone else was doing it, and having built up that love over a period of a couple of years through River, when i lost <u>him</u>, i lost all that love, and couldn't find it anywhere else.*

Years later Emma recalls feeling as a teenager that her life was unbearable. Something had to change, which is where River Phoenix came in. She remembers the warmth of 'having company' while he was in her mind, and, when she lost this through his death, this cosiness was replaced by a determination to starve herself:

'I'd always wanted to control food, to eat less, but I didn't have the willpower. I didn't have the strength. And when River Phoenix died, it became the reason why I would be able to stop eating.

'I had this safe little dream-world where things were perfect, everything was fine. And then suddenly someone came along and smashed it up and said you can't have that either. And then, I thought, "OK, I'll have nothing."'

So, this is how Emma, as a fifteen-year-old, began her journey towards clinical anorexia. She found something at last that was hers, under her command, which did not make her feel bad and inadequate but which achieved the opposite.

Control of her appetite is the first thing in her life which makes her feel good about herself. And, as she comes to realise, she would never again feel this good. For on this first hurtle down through the numbers on the weighing scale, Emma manages to starve herself for seven months.

In that time she does not deviate, look up, down, or to the side. Nor can she repeat it. It is her transcendant attempt, her most devoted and she will never do it this well again.

# Chapter Fourteen

## SLIDING DOWN

Little attention has been paid to Emma's appearance over the years and, along with much else, she has hidden her distress about it. Occasionally, as a child, she spoke angrily of her sticky-out ears. But she was not interested in my responses. Emma said nothing positive about herself.

Since she seemed to care so little, I sometimes remarked on her silky hair, how lovely her skin was, or the pretty colour of a cardigan. Or I might pick out a pattern on a dress she was wearing and, running my finger over it, say how much I liked it.

'Stoical' is the best word to describe her reaction to these compliments, Emma putting up with them as if they were one of my more unfortunate foibles.

'Now can we get on with something that matters,' she seemed to be saying.

Having no idea what lay beneath Emma's seeming

indifference to her appearance, I was startled by the hidden nature – deliberate concealment? – of her natural prettiness. Difficult to describe how she managed to hide or disregard this as a child but, in some sense, she ignored her physical self, as if her body were merely some impersonal vehicle for moving about in. She seemed not to notice or care much what she wore or what she looked like.

Her disinterest in external mirrors I put down to how she was, like that. But the way she looks does matter to Emma, as her diaries, written while she is on the Unit, reveal.

*i feel like an ugly, putrid mess of fat and bone; spots and haywire hair; sticky-out ears and bulgy eyes; yellowed rotting teeth . . .*

*I'm on the train and can see the white handles of my ears ridiculously demanding attention . . . I see the apparently thin and downturned line of my lips, their miserable sullen dullness the perfect accompaniment to the foolishness of my ears.*

Later she reflects:

*My parents never recognised the things that for me were <u>achievements</u>. I was praised for the things that came naturally to me, like my intelligence, but when i really put all my effort into looking nice (<u>trying</u> to), it went unrecognised. No one ever told*

*me i looked pretty or nice, or that i was a beauti-*
*ful person (to them) and i needed them to . . .*
  *Carol gave me praise + love for being me, being*
*musical, being funny, and would often compliment my*
*appearance – but as she was the only one it was*
*coming from, i couldn't accept it, i thought she was*
*just biased.*

She writes of not knowing about make-up, where to buy clothes, how to 'put herself together' and 'make herself right' for public consumption. She was held back and unpossessed of what she felt she needed, a small 'i' on the page.

River's death changed this. Emma had a secret grief to play out and was suddenly resolute, with something important to get on with. Swiftly she moved from a held-back condition of uncertainty into a purposeful state of decision-making, starvation in mind.

I saw a lot of Emma in those months. Her weight speeding downwards, her mood, by contrast, rising, the euphoria I dreaded had returned. Along with the fake Emma, the larger than life, older version, was trying to fool us all with her elation and lies.

During this spring of her sixteenth year, Emma would have me believe she was being open and expansive, curled up on one armchair, me on another. She said she had been going through a bad time (no mention of River) and had gained a lot of weight through comfort eating. Now she

was feeling better about herself, she was tackling the
weight problem and feeling good about it.

Any particular reason for the change? I asked.

A shrug from her and a shake of her head.

In just a few weeks of visiting me, the weight was dropping off Emma at an alarming rate. Within a month or so
it was clear this was no ordinary diet. She was dangerously
out of balance.

Warning her she was losing weight too fast, Emma was
not prepared to take heed. She appeared to listen to advice
about the importance of giving her body time to adjust, of
a gradual weight-loss being a better strategy. She would even
nod from time to time, or look mildly surprised by something that was said. But this was Emma putting on a front,
and I began to feel uncomfortable and manipulated, even.
Trying to get her to eat, she would deftly turn it back on me:

'You have one,' she would say in an indulgent voice when,
hoping to tempt her, I would offer her a home-made scone.
When I tried to insist she would shrug, turn away or tell
me she wasn't hungry.

But she was. In between words as she was talking, or
when silent, listening to me, I noticed how she moved her
mouth: small movements, as if eating invisibly, something
succulent on the inside.

And in the sunny place, the kitchen, where we baked
together years ago and made cakes for her to take home
– there were tussles:

'A cup of tea?'

'No, thank you.'

'I've got herbal kinds: comfrey, camomile.'

A shake of her head.

'Juice, then?'

'Ugh, no.'

'Water?'

A downward glance and no more.

Trying to get her to face what was happening to her body, I suggest weighing her fortnightly which, to my surprise, she agrees to. But she does not seem to accept, or care about, the numbers.

'You've lost eight pounds in two weeks, Emma. What's going on?'

Silence.

'Are you eating?'

'Yes, I've been doing more exercise, that's the reason.' Or it might be she would blame the scales. 'Have you checked them lately?' she would ask complacently.

The figures continued to hurtle down, past nine stone, towards eight. Four or five stone lost in a matter of months, I warn her then: 'Emma, if you get below eight stone, I'm going to ring your mother and Paul. I have no choice. Either you eat, or we have to get medical help.'

Angrily, she glares at me. 'What do you mean, medical help?'

'I mean this big a weight-loss this fast is dangerous.'

I don't say the word 'anorexia', but on the phone, a couple of days later, I do to Paul, who takes her to the doctor.

In the week or two before I next see Emma it is clear she has gone over a line. Eight stone left behind, she is heading downwards past seven and a half, but her doctor has said he can see no particular problem with her eating. So, she has fooled him.

I ask my own GP if she will see Emma, just for one visit, for a second opinion.

Emma goes for the appointment on her own – a mistake, perhaps. On the phone afterwards, she says the doctor is going to refer her to a specialist. She is low, subdued, as if something has been taken from her.

Emma has kept herself away from me as she has gone through puberty, put on weight and conjured her affair with River Phoenix. But in the giddiness of her new-found determination to starve herself she has come back. Perhaps to be stopped, or to be applauded for her willpower: maybe both.

Able to subdue her appetite at last, a part of her wanted my approval, which I withheld. And, as her illness and confusion took deeper hold, she seemed to want to overtake or overpower me.

In her mind, we were, perhaps, in competition and, as with her anorexic friend, Katherine, who died, Emma wanted to be best: the best anorexic; the best grown-up.

Remembering her turning round and round in my hallway as a child giddy with the delight of a big, long stay, I think of her, excited and heady now, saying: 'Look, I can fly.'

And, as the person who had 'grown her fast', done the

damage of speeding her on through childhood, I put on the brakes.

How awful for her, to have me bring her down. Ground her. Now she shuts me out again.

That summer, I hear she is badly ill. In the 'best' period of starvation she writes of in her diaries, she has dropped to just above five and a half stone, and has been hospitalised.

Rushing to see her, in dread of being too late, of finding her in a coma, I stop at the end of the corridor where I am told she will be. Trying to prepare myself, I don't want my face to give me away, for her to see me shocked or, worse, flinching.

From her place in a sunny open-plan ward, in the end bed facing the corridor, she can see me approach – and our eyes meet some twenty or thirty feet off.

Her bones seem too thin to support her and her head looks huge on top of her body, her eyes too. Deliberately, she shifts her gaze from mine, turns away, back to the girl she is talking to in the bed next door.

# Chapter Fifteen

~§

## OUT ON HER OWN

During this first episode of anorexia at the age of fifteen, Emma dislikes being in the hospital she is taken to for she suffers the indignity, in her terms, of being put on a children's ward.

She knows that in some ways she is old beyond her years and deliberately starving herself for seven months doesn't seem like child's play to her. Not that she is talking about what she has done – and I do not find the words to ask.

One of the first things I learn about anorexia is what it does to ordinary language, not in the person who is ill, but in the visitor. The imploring and ordinary questions: 'why?'; 'how?'; 'what for?' cannot be spoken in the face of someone who looks as if she has emerged from Belsen.

Emma's head is vast, the bones in her arms and legs like sticks, and her eyes are unfathomable to me, hostile, even, as if she has removed herself to a place where I cannot reach her – somewhere I cannot know.

I am set back on myself, therefore, for she seems like a grey-faced ascetic elder. I feel I am being escorted round her domain by an ancient doge who, having withdrawn from the daily pettinesses of life, is privately dismissive of my prosaic and worldly concerns.

I ask if she is cold, sitting in a short-sleeved shift, and shall I get her a cardigan. She is not cold, I am informed. She does not feel the cold.

As she escorts me round the hospital at this level, high up on the fifth floor, telling me where things are, showing me an art room and letting me know she is looking forward to doing art therapy, I am at a loss.

She fails to see who I am, even, for her eyes do not, will not, take me in. Instead they transmit a powerful message. She is like a billboard flashing, starkly: 'Keep Out'.

At other times, though, the message slips and I see the girl I know, whom I have enjoyed over the years, laughed with, cared for, and I want to weep. How did we all, all the people in her life, let her come to this: this alienation; this terrible and monumental travesty?

I am angered by Emma's illness, I discover, the abandonment of flesh like a wilful desertion of what is ordinary and alive. In its place a display of bonework, something you feel you should not see, the movement, the workings, of bones. I feel voyeuristic even glancing at her body.

And then there is her awful greyness, her skin, too, starved of nourishment and air. Her illness unnerves and appals me.

I see Emma every few days for the weeks she is in this hospital, and the meetings vary. Sometimes she is herself and at others not. Sometimes she is pleased to see me, sometimes I feel like an intruder in her shut-down world. Having someone her own age as a visitor is what she likes best and if a schoolfriend arrives, I leave them to it.

I try and avoid being there the same time as Colleen, for it is awkward. By this time neither of us can work out what to say to the other and neither of us is one for small talk.

On the one occasion we are present together, sitting facing each other at either side of the bed, Emma in between, we discuss what is going to happen when Emma is discharged.

Colleen talks, in practical terms, about her coming home with an eating plan which the hospital will put together for her from which Emma will gradually gain weight and get well again. She will be healthy enough to go back to school in the autumn term and will see friends in the school summer holiday, which is about to start.

I notice Emma looking doubtful, despondent even, and I suggest she could probably do with some psychotherapy, someone she can talk to in private about her feelings. Emma looks interested, but Colleen is dead against it. Paul asks her what *she* would like.

Emma opts for therapy, which she will be able to begin

almost straight away and continue as an out-patient after she leaves. Though, as it turns out she does not stay the course with psychotherapy.

While she is still hospitalised, I take Emma out for strengthening walks, for her muscles have been under-used for a long time. She is sometimes breathless, I notice with concern, and there are other changes in her, either through a nerve which therapy touches, or through her illness, or both, which make her, quite often, disagreeable to be with.

She is curt, angry, aggressive even, and I feel as I did the year previously when she was visiting me at the house and losing weight rapidly, that she wants her will to dominate mine. If I ask how she is, how things are going, she turns this back on me with daunting and rather imperious phrases.

'And tell me, how are things in *your* life?'

In between this stonewalling behaviour, and when walking towards her, I catch glimpses of the Emma I have known for many years. Seeing her, sometimes, standing or sitting apart, a waif is what she seems like then: lost rather than withdrawn; distressed rather than angry, and I am torn, as I will be so often, in my feelings and behaviour towards her. Part of me wants to rush to her, hold her and say:

'Look, we'll get you through this. You can do it. I promise.'

Another part of me recognises the severity of her illness, the deep unhappiness she carries in her from childhood, and the long, hard work it will take to turn her towards life again.

By the early autumn of her release from hospital, Emma

is sixteen, and she, Paul and Colleen move home, leaving the flat they were in for a big house with a garden. Although three or four miles away from where they were before, Emma goes to the same school for what will be her last year.

While I am relieved at the amount of space there is, the house is old and neglected, with bare boards in most of the rooms, and it is cold. When I visit her Emma looks frail, wears long loose flapping clothes, and her hands are icy.

That autumn term, Emma sits mock GCSEs. Having lost a lot of time, she is nervous. She is also a perfectionist, which only increases her anxiety about how well she will do. In a number of long phone conversations, I reassure her about what she *does* know, how capable she is and how these exams will be well within her reach.

And she does marvellously, phones in January to say she has got mainly As and is expected to do possibly even better in June for the 'real thing'.

Glad for her, glad, too, to hear the vibrancy and strength in her voice, I am also troubled. By this time Emma has gained weight again. Until around Christmas, this had been reassuring. It might suggest anorexia is a one-off episode. But by the following spring she is getting heavy, around eleven to twelve stone and looking gorgeous as she so easily does. But, Emma's weight gain is too much and too fast.

Emma becomes increasingly euphoric; bursts of elation include excited talk of buying furniture for her room (which she does not have the money for), and travelling the world. But she is also what I can only describe as over-contained.

No one else is in any of her plans, I notice, and I wonder how to find a way of influencing these dangerous traits without bringing Emma down. She and her illness are so intertwined it is difficult to get at one without the other. And, as before, Emma says nothing about her dramatic gain in weight. Like a vessel travelling full-steam ahead, she gives the impression of heeding no one outside herself and I fear there will be no turning her.

This fear, however, is overtaken by another crisis. Suddenly, Emma becomes terrified of her impending exams. Talking to her mother about it, Colleen has said she should wait, not put herself through the strain. She has missed time, after all, and could take her GCSEs the following year.

I feel this would be disastrous for her. Emma is one of the oldest in her class anyway. If she stays back a year, she will be almost eighteen, all her friends will have moved on, and she will feel left behind and unmotivated. I say I will help her through. We will do some revision and home-work together and it will not matter, in any case, what the results are. She should forget about those. Just sit the exams. Just do it.

I remember these times vividly, walking together in a park near to where she has moved, me imploring, exhort-ing her not to give up:

'They're not important, these exams. In themselves, they're nothing. It's just that, without them, you will be on one side of a closed door and the opportunity to do what you want with your life will be on the other.

'Then you'll have to knock hard – and it will be boring. You will get very bored. Why not just walk through?'

I am concerned about pushing Emma. To a friend who asks about her one day I hear myself say, wearily:

'Well, I'm frogmarching her through GCSEs.' This is what it feels like, that I am marching her through, against her will. But where is Emma's will by this time?

The exam results, a few months later, are marvellous: eight GCSEs, many of them starred 'As'. But Emma is in free-fall, increasingly unrealistic, unaware of other people. It is obvious, as it has been for some time, that she is ill again, her eating out of control.

Emma's weight, from when she left hospital the previous summer to sitting GCSEs in June 1995, has almost doubled, from around seven to almost thirteen stone.

So her control of food after the death of River Phoenix had failed, utterly, to subdue her craving. Instead, carnivore-like, her appetite has roared back at her, hunting her down, making her once more a slave to binge-eating.

# Chapter Sixteen

❧

## LYME REGIS

When asked, years later, why her GCSEs were such a struggle and why she almost refused to take them, Emma said she was ashamed to go to school and be seen by people:

'My eating was out of control, but I wouldn't admit it. I knew I was gaining weight all the time and I was very ashamed about it. I was greedy – and I couldn't stop it. So I felt I was a terrible person.

'I didn't want anyone to see me. I was completely miserable – and very angry, I realise. Lots of anger inside me.'

During this time, Emma went through a gothic phase that lasted a year or two. She says she found in punk and the culture which surrounded it an expression for her anger. Having done little with her appearance, now she began to colour her golden-brown hair mixtures of dark red and black. She wore black clothes, black nail varnish and lipstick. She looked striking. A statuesque girl with beautiful fair colouring, large eyes, luscious skin, and all this black. I thought of saying something, for she wore tight black mini-skirts with black fishnet tights, and was noticed wherever she went. But then at her age, or slightly older, I was wearing a beehive hairdo, green eyeshadow, stiletto heels and skirts, or pelmets, which were even shorter. So, I kept my mouth shut.

As with her large weight gains, Emma seemed oblivious of the effect her appearance had on people around her. It was not what the clothes were for, to attract attention or to show rebellion, but rather to keep people away, to provide her with a defence. She wanted to be impervious, out on her own, sailing solo.

That September, with Emma in full goth mode, she and I went to the small seaside town of Lyme Regis. With its centuries-old harbour and stone cob made famous by *The French Lieutenant's Woman*, she had heard me talk of it many times one of my favourite places to go. It was her reward for taking GCSEs. She could have money, or a treat, I had said.

Choosing the latter she said she wanted time away with me, to walk by the sea, hear the gulls, the waves, feel the wind in her hair. So, setting off in the car, Lyme Regis it was.

But only just. For Emma's appearance – coupled with her extraordinary way of shutting people out – was, in this small town, out of season, visitors gone, something to behold and be wary of.

The third time a B and B 'Vacancies' sign was flipped over it became obvious it was Emma, or the apparition of her slowly following me, that was causing this turn-around. We even had a room once.

'Oh, yes,' the landlady said brightly as I asked for a twin-bedded. Then, as Emma arrived in the doorway: 'Actually, I believe we're fully booked . . .'

'They're nervous of how you look,' I said, with a smile.

Shrugging her shoulders, she said nothing.

So, keeping her safely in the car, I went to an old creaky hotel, long-since closed, paid for a twin room up front, and in she came.

Her memories of that time are of being cold. She had not brought a warm coat, had refused the offer of one of mine, so we walked in blustery weather, her in thin clothes and only a cardigan.

She did not complain. In fact, said practically nothing all weekend. Except for the Saturday evening when, sitting in a harbour pub having a meal, a couple nearby began to talk to us.

Having recently moved into the town, there were plenty of business opportunities, they said, lots of money to be made. They did go on a bit. After a while it was Emma who said:

'Carol writes books.'

A pause, a brief question about what kind of books, and a return to talk of business. Leaving soon after, me saying wryly they were obviously not the reading kind, Emma replied: 'They're jealous of you.'

'Why?'

'Because you're real.'

Would she be up for a hug I wondered, but her expression remained serious, the 'Keep Out' message securely in place. No more was said that night. My wish to get her to talk, to melt, thwarted, we returned to the hotel in silence.

Lying in bed, trying to sleep, there were noises all round: creaking floorboards and doors; ancient plumbing; voices. Then there was Emma. Restless, awake, she shuffled, moved, tossed, turned, sighed, got up, went out, came back, went out again, sighed, shuffled, tossed, turned. Asking if she was all right, there was silence, and then a low, controlled: 'Yes. I don't want to keep you awake.'

Pretending to sleep, I lay exhausted, as Emma's what? – her distress? – went on through the night. Did she sleep at all? I wondered. She looked drained in the morning.

'You didn't sleep well?' I half asked.

'I've got a heavy period and was afraid of getting the sheets stained.'

'We could have bought something yesterday. I could have helped.'

A shake of her head. 'I've got things with me. I was just afraid.'

It took me years to realise what her awful secret was that night. Food. Under the bedclothes, in the corridor, unwrapping chocolate wrappers and crisp packets in the loo, bringing food back to bed, going out to unwrap more, Emma was eating in the dark.

I thought I could hear rustlings, and decided I was imagining it. But there it was, Emma at her most driven, compulsive, desperate: and me, literally, in the dark.

At the pub the previous night, her way with food was, as it had always been in public, dispassionate. Showing no interest in the menu or, eventually, in the food on her plate, she sat with me as I enjoyed eating as if I, again, were the prosaic person governed by appetite and she removed from such mundane matters.

Indulgent with me as I lingered clearing my plate, Emma was waiting patiently for later when she would eat out of sight and under her control, in the hotel corridor and beneath the bedclothes. Then, as always, she chose snacky things: chocolate bars, crisps and biscuits.

Knowing that in Emma's life at this time, and for some years to come, her illness was what she had, I can see why she wanted to keep it – and keep it secret. For who would she be, stripped of it? In bondage to the sweet things she thought she could never get enough of, Emma's outward presentation, the persona she gave the world, was therefore daunting.

Her way of rebuffing people who might have questioned her food habits was almost masterly. The impression she gave was of immense privacy, as if guarding something of great personal value.

I thought she was trying to grow up, that she was making a stand against authority and letting me know not to spoil it for her.

Trying to devise possible routes through her guarded lines that she would not resent or feel invaded by made me feel like a burglar, a thief, and it is not that way round.

The *unpossession* in Emma, the knowledge she, herself, has not taken and grasped from childhood, which she has in a sense 'stolen' from her life, is manifest on the return journey to London. We hit a bad traffic jam on the M3, stopping and starting every few hundred yards. I ask Emma to get a large easy-to-read map from the back seat and plan us a route back to London, ideally by getting off at the next turning.

She glares at me.

'What's wrong?'

'I don't know what you mean,' she says, in a strained, controlled voice, and then, almost angrily: 'I don't know what you want.'

Explaining that I want her to look up Winchester in the index, I say she will then find the M3 and London on the same page. Then it is a question of finding a road off the M3 that leads towards London.

This frightens her, as I afterwards realise, and as I glance at her struggling with it, I see the atlas is beyond her – a closed book. Not because she is not capable of this, but because she is at a loss. The key to this map, and many others, is one she has not picked up.

Emma's weight will climb a little more after this.

Then, in the winter after her seventeenth birthday, as she

attends Sixth Form College and begins an A-level course, it will suddenly plummet again – numbers tumbling down the scales, pounds and stones dropping away.

# Chapter Seventeen

## A Big Relationship

Emma's sense of herself, of who she is, what she is good at, seemed to be almost non-existent. Before beginning her A-level course, she had no idea which subjects to take, or what degree she might be interested in. A dilemma faced by many students, in Emma it was acute.

Talking about it in my flat, we ranged over a large area of possibilities. She clearly loved the arts: music; art; photography. Would she like to study something she was passionate about, I asked her, or would she prefer to make a different kind of career choice?

She seemed to like computers. She could do something like Information Technology or Computer Graphics. Would she like to be a librarian of some kind?

Not wanting to 'steer' Emma in this important choice, wanting it to be hers, she disconcertingly keeps on passing it back to me. She is not sure what to do for the best. What do I think?

Well she is good, more than good, at art, photography, design, music, English, more or less equally. But it is her future, her life we are discussing. Where does her passion lie? What does Emma love?

In a few years' time she will be able to tell me. Singing will be one of her favourite things to do. Art, photography, music of many kinds she will also deeply enjoy. But for now?

Emma decides to take A-level Art; Philosophy, because she is interested in thinking about the world and how it works; and Music Technology. It seems a good choice to me.

For the next year or more, while she is at her parents' home and studying for A-levels, I see little of Emma: around three or four visits, that is all. When we see each other, her weight has continued to rise – to above thirteen stone – but I feel I can say nothing.

Phoning her from time to time, she seems to be studying and going out with friends. In some senses, then, being a typical teenager.

Thinking about her, as I do, trying to be optimistic, I tell myself Sixth Form College will involve her in interesting work. In giving her a fresh start, she will have the chance to gain confidence and meet new people. She will perhaps find someone, a friend or a teacher, who will warm to her, discern the shy, afraid-to-ask child through the contained, imposing and seemingly impervious girl.

But I am fooling myself. Emma comes to see me in the

second term of her course, saying she wants to drop two A-levels, to spend the remainder of her time – eighteen months – studying just Art.

Not realising the full extent of her return to her illness by this point, I am, initially, hard on her. Why only one A-level? I ask. Why can't she manage more? Is it the work itself that's too much? Is it the teaching? Does she need help of some kind?

Emma can only tell me she cannot do it and, after a while, I see there is no point in going further. Her voice is husky, almost breaking. She is clearly distressed.

'I'd hoped you'd understand,' she says.

I don't.

'You know I'd never want you to do what's beyond you. But you won't get on a good university course with one A-level.'

She looks wretched, and I add: 'If it would make you ill to do more, then obviously you musn't.'

But as she heads into the winter preceding her A-level, she is secretly vomiting again, binge-purging, and there is room in her life for little else. The long loop which will bring her crashing down for the second time has begun. I, certainly, am to be avoided.

Keeping away from me for most of the time she is at Sixth Form College is something Emma does deliberately. Writing of it in her diaries, and speaking to me later, she says:

'I wanted to push you away because I knew that if I let you, you would help me. I knew you would know there was something wrong – and you would try and do something about it. I didn't want that. I had to have my illness. I was so unhappy. I had to have something.'

The 'something' is a 'big' relationship, which Emma yearns to engage with, to have all to herself and to keep close to her, in contrast to the real world where friendships and life itself have always been difficult.

The serious nature of the first long loop of her illness has not changed Emma or her world as she must have hoped it would. It has not brought her the insights and the authority she wished for.

For Emma is searching for something. She is, I believe, looking for meaning, for identity, for the remembered and ingested nature of an experience that will stay with her. Build her up.

She wants something she can accrue, which will be hers to have and to call on, and which will not desert her:

*Eating out of desperation – what else can I do? It's my only available comfort, my solace, my lover and friend . . . The craving mounts with every mouthful of sweetness – every morsel i consume is to fuel the fire of my longing . . . is there any more?*

Years later, I can understand Emma keeping all this from

me, for of course I would have intervened. And it is not
possible to say, now, whether that would have been a good
or a bad thing. For anorexia was, for Emma, a necessity.
It was *her* way. And, as her teenage years became more
and more bleak and removed from reality, it was not her
only abuse.

Under an entry which begins 'i am a liar', there is a
headline MY PAST in which she writes of these sixth-form
years:

> i drank a bottle of vodka and took a handful of
> Pro-Plus tablets, and stayed out all night.
>     I bought my first bottle of vodka in the summer
> of 1995. In the house i'd have music on, windows
> wide open, and i'd sing loudly and drink vodka and
> orange. From then until my bulimia started again
> at the end of 1996 i made sure that there was
> always a bottle of vodka at the ready. Some days i
> needed to drink before i could leave the house, meet
> friends, go to college . . .

So, this is what Emma was hiding, and why she could not
manage to take three A-levels. Bulimia already threatening
again, she was engaged elsewhere and way out of control:

> Summer 1996 – Pro-Plus, music on, curtains closed,
> dancing + dancing to techno upstairs in my room.
> i'd go out to clubs with Ellen. We'd be drunk on

*vodka and i'd pretend to have taken something, E or speed. Sometimes i'd pretend to be out of it when we were together so that i'd be more interesting. Sometime i'd act spacey in front of my parents to make them think i was doing normal teenage things. i'd do things to make them think i had a boyfriend too . . .*

   *I'm a liar — i've never taken <u>LOADS</u> of drugs never taken acid, or loads of Es, never had an <u>actual</u> drug problem except from the one in my head.*

Emma's diaries tell us that food is her 'voice', the way she speaks to herself, her central and overwhelming relationship.

However, Emma did not want anorexia to kill her, any more than she wanted to hate her mother. She had not set out to be hating and hateful, nor to die, but to find a different way: to escape what she felt to be the badness, the meaninglessness and the guilt of her life.

And life itself, the rainbow life, is an image she was still drawn to and reaching out for, for Emma's relationship with anorexia had chinks in it. She longed for those bits of real life which had come to matter to her and which, perhaps, brought her peace:

*if i were a colour i'd wish to be white. Forever clean, pure, honest and serene. In reality i imagine that i'm more of a rainbow, more colourful that i wish or admit to be . . . if I were a building i'd be a library. Quiet, filled with stories, surprises and things of interest waiting to be drawn out and discovered and enjoyed by other people.*

*A library waits to be discovered.*

But anorexia, so engrossing and overwhelming, was something she wanted more than anything or anyone else.

She has written that her first episode was like a fog and she decides she wants to repeat her illness, in order, she rationalises, to remember it, to *have* it this time round.

# Chapter Eighteen

❧

## UNPLACED LOVE

After a period of bingeing, Emma begins to starve herself again, ending up in a local hospital when she is just turned eighteen. Sent home after a long weekend of being drip-fed, she hovers, for a number of months, at just below seven stone, and then another drop.

I discover from Emma's diaries that by the following year she is less than six stone, and has been referred to the Unit for a month, the place where I eventually catch up with her in 1998.

Seeing her rarely, I am unaware of this first stay on the Unit. Beds are short at that time too, as they are when I visit her almost exactly a year later, and she is discharged after four weeks, to attend sessions as a day-patient while she lives at home.

Visiting her there Emma seems somewhat better, although rather subdued. And there is good news: she has won a place at the Guildhall in London to study art and design.

Knowing how much her artwork means to her, I hope this is the breakthrough which will bring Emma out of her self-imposed cocoon. If she could step into life, become a student, open herself up to possibilities, she might stop being overwhelmed by the pain of her past.

But I have not seen enough of her of late fully to realise how far beneath the surface Emma has gone. The outside world is an alien and distant place for her with its demands, immediacies and jagged edges and she cannot sustain herself there.

> *There's an argument going on inside my head – should i or should i not go down to the kitchen and binge? [purge]. It's the feeling that i desperately don't want to do it that's making me want to – it feels like i can't go to sleep without having done something nasty to myself.*

The ugliness that I often see in Emma's illness is present in the feelings she has about herself. In the mirror inside Emma sees someone who deserves to be harmed, and she writes of her wish to disfigure herself, to make the world see the same painful picture:

> *I <u>want</u> to make myself vomit – continue to rot my teeth, unbalance my potassium levels, get dizzy*

*spells, get mouth ulcers which often develop into large bubbles of blood that i burst . . . i want to pick my skin until it bleeds and then scabs over, and scars . . . I'm glad that i'm making myself ugly. . . I want to see how much pain i can cause myself and how disgusting i can make myself look . . .*

*i despise myself . . . i feel like a real nuisance . . . I know i need to be looked after at the moment . . . but i don't know how to accept support without feeling greedy . . . I've run back to my bulimia because it's safe. This is a painful choice too, but it's a path i can comprehend + control, unlike my emotions which keep on overwhelming me.*

This inner sense of self-loathing influences how Emma behaves: sometimes lashing out at people; at others pleading for help.

As usual, there are signposts pointing both ways, with despair and determination to self-harm followed by times where she thinks she might like to be well. But for months she is bleak:

*It's sunny, but i can't feel any warmth, only the chill . . .*
*Sometimes i think the coldness comes from within me, and everyone is actually warmed, except me.*

*I don't know how to get through my sadness, my pain, my unplaced love.*

Coming across these last two words, reading them six or seven years on, I stop for a long time. In a sense, they say it all. No wonder she felt cold inside, held back and uncertain.

For who, where, was she without her love?

In the many reasons for Emma's illness: her difficult childhood; her strong will; her sensitive, talented and addictive nature; this would seem to come first, a feeling of her love not mattering.

Unplaced, it left Emma without a radiating way of giving out and bringing back affection, friendship, life. Unable to take, to give, and to find where her passions lay, so much in Emma was unearthed: music; art; friendships; her parents; me; and most of all herself.

Self-denial and, eventually, self-harm, took the place of the warmth and care for herself which her *placed*, possessed – and valued – love may have provided.

Failing to take up her place at Guildhall in the autumn of 1997 Emma says, on the phone, she does not feel well enough to do it and can say no more.

*my head is so full i feel . . . i'm going completely mad. i feel so much like 2 different people that i can have a running dialogue in my mind with both sides: Emma the sadist; emma the victim.*

*As well as these 2, theres also Me, my intel-
ligence + rational mind which refuses to take sides
. . .*

*i'm losing track of the days, of all sense of time,
as well as my sense of purpose. What the fuck do
i think i'm doing?*

*i feel like i've stepped into a surreal nightmare
world, and i keep wanting to just take off + run
away from it all. But i don't have anywhere to run
to. i don't want to be on the Unit, or at home, or
at a friends house, or out, or in, with people,
alone, awake, asleep —*

*i've felt this way before, when i was on my
own with bulimia before i'd even heard of the
Unit. This overwhelming feeling inside, forebod-
ing, doom — a sense that something enormous is
going to rise up and devour me. its like a coil
inside, getting tighter and tighter wound, only a
matter of time before it lets go and explodes. i'm
so frightened, but i don't know what of.*

My re-entry into Emma's life begins with a phonecall. Her
soft voice tells me she is ill, in hospital, and wants me to
visit. Little more is said.

The call does not surprise me, I notice, as if I have been
waiting a long, long time – years – for it to happen. And
how brave of her to ring.

She must have known I would ask a lot of her, that with

the knowledge of her past, and the skills at my disposal,
I would question, as well as care for her, would implore
her towards living.

In a sense, I had never made it easy for Emma to avoid
life. Courageous then, for her to bring me back in.

# Chapter Nineteen

## LIVING WITH GHOSTS

Emma thinks she may be missing something. There is something vital she has to have, wants to see and experience, before she leaves what she describes as the 'cold hallways' of anorexia behind. For, to her mind, there may still be something there, in the illness, which she has not quite grasped:

> i want to kiss the bottom of the ocean before i burst through its surface into the sunlight. Otherwise i'll always be wondering about what was left unseen at its bottom.

So, despite starving herself three times, once, as she writes, for those first seven months straight through, Emma is still on the look-out for an unclaimed experience on the ocean floor of anorexia.

It is not just quantity she wants from her illness – time: weeks, months, to stay in it as she wishes – but also 'quality': something of value which might be hers to claim. Rather than risk leaving this elusive prize behind, she will think of diving once more.

She has written about it, often, that she wants *all* of anorexia. Some of it is not enough:

> i fully intend to see it through . . . to the point where i can pause and know that i've gone far enough, that i've done it.

Further on in this passage is the place where Emma writes of 'harnessing death and choosing life'. Hers is not a suicide quest but a wish for the kind of power and superiority not available to the rest of us – to hover near death, see it and be able to choose to leave it behind.

> how many steps from death must i get before i decide that i don't want to die . . . ?
>
> Anorexia has been the shadowy figure in my past, a clean and noble ghost hovering over me . . . The elegant grace of the pale, thin, empty body . . . i want to keep existing in this for a while, because unless i do, i know that i'll always have a secret yearning for anorexia . . .
>
> look how skinny . . . my body a landscape of jutting bone and painful recesses. See my deathly

*pallor, the light of the lie of life in my dying
eyes . . . see me wearing death and cloaking myself
in this deep heady promise of safety and control
and comfort.*

High romance, baroque teenage fantasy perhaps, and yet on reading her diaries I continue to question why, how, did it lead to this, and why does it continue?

She was once a child painting pictures in my living room and listening to stories, curled round me, head in my lap. Now there is ambivalence and a struggle in her with me around. Head, face pulled from side to side sometimes, as if I am here and the hypnotic gaze of her mirror-friend there, she is torn between the two of us. Yet, whatever calls anorexia makes on her to deny me, she continues to allow me in.

Sitting still in the armchair opposite, I see in Emma the ghosts of her coffins, hallways and beckoning friends. I glimpse the path of her illness: Emma a thoroughfare for life, death and the wraiths which pull her about.

Standing or sitting at times like this, Emma says nothing, and I wait a while until she turns back to me, naked, deserted. All of them gone.

If only she would say the words 'Help me.' Her shoulders, her eyes do, her face does, but her arms stay by her side. It is always *me* who reaches for *her*.

Sometimes, though, seeing the effort it costs Emma, this struggle, I leave her go, let her be. I know I must not, cannot, challenge her too much and too far. It would be too big a strain for her and might break her will instead of her illness. And she needs her will to fight if she is prepared to do so.

If I am to understand Emma's alienating, killing preoccupation I will have to be patient. As Emma has to be, her own form of painstaking attention wrought over years of living with her illness:

> i need to move very slowly . . . i'm going to get to a point where my body frightens me – when it becomes a fully functioning body again, womanly and alive and real. It _will_ repulse me, and i _will_ want to hurt it. It's going to be extremely difficult and i'll need a lot of help + support when this happens. i think i'll need my bulimia again at this stage, or else i'll probably return to my compulsive eating which feels completely out of control and compounds my feelings of greed and laziness.

Visiting her, seeing her regularly, I sense Emma spends much of her time somewhere else, removed from the world where I live my life, and I cannot just drag her away from this inner place where she feels she belongs.

She has lived more of her life here, among her ghosts, wraiths, mirror-friends than with me, or with anyone else. It is her home.

Emma's lies emerge at this stage, about whether she is eating or not; about what she does during the day; and over things like arrangements for meetings – with Therese, for example.

Both with busy lives, Therese and I have already got into a mess over a changed appointment time which, it turns out, Emma was supposed to tell me about. Then there is the all-important case meeting to discuss what will happen to Emma when she leaves the Unit for good in a few weeks' time.

From the staff's point of view, she has made good progress: both in terms of a weight gain of over a stone since she was admitted less than two months ago; and her positive response to the various therapies. She is judged to have the beginning of an understanding of her illness and, through this, the means to begin to manage on her own.

But, talking to me that morning, before we go into the meeting, Emma is tense, edgy, almost despairing. While staff on the Unit might have faith in her, she has little in herself. And there is still nowhere for her to live. For Emma, home with Colleen and Paul remains a place of either over-eating or under-eating.

I, too, have been a pain in her terms. I have pushed the issue of her not taking my help and me seriously. When asked about me, she continues with the 'Oh, Carol's a friend' tag, refusing to acknowledge publicly how close we are, and I fear this will have practical consequences. Knowing how systems work and the strains they are under,

I sense I will have to stand up for her. Yet how can I do this convincingly when Emma, as an adult, is not convinced herself?

Unofficial godmother is a tag I come up with to get us through the business of my having a place in her life. Reluctantly, as if I am being a nuisance and she has no idea why I am making such a fuss about it, Emma agrees.

By the time we go into the case meeting which will begin to shape the rest of Emma's life, she and I are both exhausted. She is panicked at the thought of leaving the Unit so soon, of being 'pushed out', as she refers to it, before she is ready. I am worried too, with things moving so fast. Just a few weeks more might make all the difference, but it is not for me to decide.

The ensuing discussion at the meeting is not easy, at least not the practical side of it. While doctors sympathetically ask Emma how she is feeling, and she gives vaguely optimistic and misleading replies about how she is ready to try and manage on her own, there is the predicted housing problem.

Therese is thinking of placing Emma in a hostel, when a room can be found. Having an inkling of what this might mean, what it might be like, I ask about smoking.

'She really hates cigarette smoke,' I say to the dozen or so people assembled.

'It's emotional as well as physical. Ever since she was a small child she's reacted to it, and if there's a lot of it in the hostel . . .'

There is an awkward silence. Therese shuffling papers, says she will look into it and can make no promises.

Emma is silent, as is the rest of the group.

Before I can stop myself I have said it:

'She can stay with me – until something more permanent is sorted out.'

A rustle of relief.

'Would you like that?' a doctor asks Emma, kindly.

'Yes,' she says, turning to me. 'Thank you.'

# Chapter Twenty

❧

## MOTHER-FOOD

Preparing for Emma's stay with me, I read a number of books on anorexia to try and understand it more and help us both with the difficult time ahead.

While most professionals in the field say there is no one root cause of the illness, one account gives a direct way of understanding what is happening between Emma and me, the way she both wants my help and refuses to accept it.

Written by a psychotherapist, Dr Gianna Williams, it describes anorexia as involving: 'impairment in "taking from another"' in 'internalising a dependent relationship'. The impaired relationship is, overwhelmingly, with the mother, but continues with other people.

Dr Williams writes that this arises from an early break in a feeding pattern between a mother and child (which can be accidental) where the child comes to reject, and to continue to reject into her teenage years, 'mother-food'; emotional and practical knowledge about daily life and the hundreds of bits of everyday learning a parent passes on to a small child.

Some of my frustration with Emma is helped by reading this. It explains her reluctance and difficulty in accepting my help. She might take it in to some extent and then reject it, vomit it up.

It makes sense, too, of her pleas about not knowing how to live her life, of not feeling competent in small everyday ways. I have been startled by the extent of her questions about aspects of daily living: how to ask for things in shops; how to choose what to wear to go out; how to use a knife and fork; to crack the top of an egg; and how to wash herself, even.

*It's not that I don't want to grow up, it's that I don't know how to.*

Having rejected 'mother-food', it is hardly surprising that Emma hungered, not only for food itself, but for the reassurance of adulthood and autonomy. Far from being on the way to achieving this by the age of nineteen, Emma is severely held back.

*i rarely felt confident that my mum loved me, when she showed that love i wanted to cling to it, prolong it, savour it because i didn't know when i'd next*

*feel it . . . i can recall doing <u>anything</u> to keep*
*her attention - if i was getting her attention when*
*i was ill then i'd really play up my illness for*
*all it was worth . . .*

*If i'm only shown a certain amount of something,*
*i feel that that's all i deserve & that i'm not*
*allowed to ask for any more than that because i feel*
*greedy.*

In reading this, the clear and heart-rending picture I have
is of Emma as a child, especially among other children,
hanging back. Not asking for more. Not daring to.

Yet, Emma says stubborn is the word most commonly used
about her behaviour with adults – that, and demanding.
She remembers wanting to be stopped from being like this,
for being indulged did not bring Emma the feeling of
belonging and ease, peace even, that she so wanted.
Instead, Colleen and Paul's seeming indifference to her
poor behaviour produced in her a feeling of deep dissatis-
faction and more craving.

I, as a source of mother-food, some of which she accepted and enjoyed as a child, failed to prevent Emma reaching for anorexia. The extent of her unhappiness and her
overwhelming feeling of ingrained badness meant she was
'bound to do something'. She says she would have turned
to drugs had they been more readily available.

With so much darkness and confusion inside her she
turned somewhere 'cleaner' and more controllable than

ordinary life: an illness where she could stop it all and be only a shadow of her former self.

In the stressful time before staying with me, Emma writes about guilt:

> i haven't grown up completely yet. There's still a small girl in my centre who believes that the world revolves around her alone and that anything and everything that takes place in the world can somehow be related directly back to her. it's from this centre that the feelings of guilt emanate . . .
>
> The small girl in my centre takes on all the pains and the mistakes of the world and is obediently willing to believe that 'it's all my fault' . . . She sometimes wonders if she's really to blame . . . but there's no one she can trust enough to give her the answer she needs to hear. She's far too afraid of having her own beliefs confirmed – that she is bad, selfish, dirty, wrong and evil.

Emma is an extraordinary mixure of vulnerability and self-will at this time, of determination and skinlessness. And, despite the books I have read, I, too, still misjudge the extent of her feeling of nakedness in the world, of her *un*possession: the effect of what she has *not* learned, *not* taken, *not* eaten:

> i'm too afraid to face the world without placing

*something between myself and it as my protection,*
*to prevent feeling exposed as my true self. When*
*this protective barrier is not my eating disorder,*
*as is currently the case, i'm in a constant state of*
*tense panic, my mind scrabbling about for something*
*else i can use as my shield.*

As with all the ambivalence her diary reveals, Emma both
wants to guard her territory, to use her defence – and to
be stopped from using it.

*i'm not stopped.*
*i want to be stopped.*

In the spaciousness of the house Emma visited as a young
child – sold a couple of years back – she could have 'got on
with' being ill. She could have withdrawn behind her
defences, beaten her fists against the wall, or stuck pins in
effigies of *me*. There would have been plenty of room for
Emma and her illness. I, too, would have had the opportunity both to relax and to prepare myself.

The flat I moved to has no such tolerance. The small
second bedroom given over to a study, Emma will have
to sleep in the living room, which is also the dining area,
which has a small kitchen leading off it. Her put-you-
up bed will be stowed behind an armchair in the corner
with the bedding on top. There will be no room for the
clutter she likes around her or for privacy for us both.

With her stay approaching, I am concerned about the arrangement and resigned, as my notes at the time reveal:

> *I couldn't see any other way* [of helping her] – *and what choice was there? Either my floor or somebody else's.*

Emma is even more fearful:

> *In a few days I go on leave for 2 weeks to stay with Carol – and I'm completely petrified.*

# Chapter Twenty-One

## EMMA'S LION

Suddenly Emma seems to be my responsibility again. I had told people at her case meeting I could offer her three or four weeks until permanent accommodation was arranged. I would be going on holiday to France at the end of June, a time when it would be easy for her to stay in an empty flat. She had visited before, I explained, and liked my home, so it was not unknown territory.

Therese is on the phone the following morning, holding me to this and more if she can. She says she wants to talk through arrangements for reviewing Emma's progress and to discuss what is to be done with her over the next month or so. She says she has organised a flat for Emma to move into, a permanent place, for about six weeks' time.

A pause.

The 'about' clangs heavily in my ears, and I resist the bait.

Which is just as well, for it will be around three months before Emma moves to a flat of her own.

I agree she can stay for the week before France, the week I am away and two weeks following. Four weeks in total.

'Any longer might strain the relationship,' I explain. 'She will, after all, be sleeping in a makeshift bed, or on cushions on the floor.'

A sigh from Therese but no 'thank you', I notice, for having bought her four weeks' grace. Instead a statement that she will, of course, be visiting Emma during the time she is in my flat to make sure the accommodation is up to standard and that Emma is happy with it.

One of the saving graces between Emma and me, even when she is ill, is a shared sense of humour. Still 'silly' after all these years, we are used to each other's wry ways and when I warn her, in mock alarm, that Therese will be on the warpath, investigating my establishment, making sure it is up to scratch, Emma smiles:

'Oh, will she,' she responds, 'I wouldn't bet on it.'

During her time with me, Emma will sleep at my place and carry on going to the Unit from Monday to Friday, between ten and six as a day-patient. There she will continue to see the friends she has made and to receive professional help.

She will see a dietician, as she has done before, and be monitored for how she is eating. She will attend planned meal-times, have individual therapy and be part of the on-going programme which has formed the basis of her recovery including art and music therapy and creative writing. So she is not without support.

Around this time, though, she writes of her inability or unwillingness to be supported, either by her peers at the Unit, or, as it will turn out, by me:

> *I started crying when the group* [therapy] *was over because the last thing we did upset me – we all held a piece of the same cloth, leaned back and supported each other's weight. I couldn't do it. I bent my legs and elbows and stood very firm, yet . . .*
>
> *I needed to feel supported, as i do in my life, but i can't let myself be, and i pretend not to need that support.*

Speaking to a friend, a film producer who has made a documentary about anorexia, I say I am concerned, with Emma being with me, that she will resent my support, that she will see my action in saving her from friends' floors as interference. Gillian thinks differently, says she believes Emma will be strengthened by my presence, by being able to lean on me for a while, possibly as someone who is a supportive mother figure but not a mother.

In the week before I help Emma move her belongings into my place, she is at her most frightened and confused.

For mothering of any kind is not what she thinks she needs. It is, in a sense, what she has spent her life fleeing from. At the same time, she has a fantasy notion of abundant, unconditional mothering which she yearns for.

Sensing some of her anxiety, I spend a lot of time talking with Emma about her stay and how it might help her. She can use me and the safety of my flat to relax and to gain strength and stability. She can go for walks along the canal, sit under the trees there, or in the garden.

Emma seems pleased with this, says it will give her time to think, to understand what she does with her eating disorder and why she continues it. She has begun to realise that she repeats certain episodes in her life which make her prone or vulnerable to her illness.

She says she does not want to 'get into the loop again of getting out, seeing people, getting speeded up, overeating, and then crashing into the buffers'. We think that being in my place, free of peer pressure, she will have a chance to find a different way.

She starts to speak of her childhood nostalgically one day, as if it is something she has missed and wants either to keep or to regain, and writes:

*I don't want to leave my whole childhood behind, but i don't know which bits of it are safe for me to keep when so much of it is so tangled up with the bad eating habits i've developed, and i've noticed that when i get nostalgic about my past, my old eating habits resurface, mostly in the urge to binge on lots of sweet, nice foods.*

However, seeing her on the Unit the day following, things are very different, the much-prized ease which Emma hopes to find with me replaced by self-denial and disgust. Pacing the room, she is distraught. I can almost see her being pulled about, consumed by self-hatred.

Taking her outside to try and walk off some demons, she tells me she is bad, evil, that she has been one long mess since childhood, that she was a bad child then, deeply flawed, and is a bad person now.

'You're not a bad person,' I implore her on a bleak roadway, leading to what looks like a brickworks at the back of the hospital.

'You're suffering an effect – and there was a cause. You're responding to a cause. There's no deep flaw in you, no fault.'

'I'm just a lump of shit. I'm not worth anything. I might as well be dead.'

'There was a reason for you to be ill,' I plead with her. 'You were deeply unhappy . . .'

'Other people are unhappy. They don't starve themselves,' she shouts.

'None of us does the same things, Emma. We have different strengths and weaknesses. That's what we try and understand in ourselves – and forgive.'

'I can't. I can't do it. I don't deserve to be alive.' Tears then, sobs, as I hold her.

See-sawing up and down, in and out of extremes of anger and acceptance, hope and despair, we visit my flat together to look at where her bed might go and to see how we will manage the space. Emma is strained.

In the middle of the afternoon, both of us sitting on the settee, it is time for her snack. In order to keep on gaining weight she eats three meals at set times at this stage and has set snack-times in between.

Getting up from the settee to fetch a small plastic bottle of juice, Emma is taut. Watching her move, she is like an addict, her focus entirely on the bottle and I cannot, for the moment, reach her or get her to recognise me. As with her first episode of anorexia, she does not seem to 'see' me. I am sitting next to her, and yet I am not part of her tightly focused world. She is obsessed and, as she writes at times in her diaries, addicted.

Slowly, at first, she begins to shake the bottle. Then faster, she shakes and shakes, over and over. After a bit, my nerves taut, I say, mildly,

'Are you going to drink it?'

She looks as if she might burst into tears. This is quickly replaced by something else – determination? – and she continues to shake, all her focus, her world at that moment, in the bottle.

As will happen on a number of occasions, I walk away. Going into the bedroom, I sit for a few minutes, to calm myself. I cannot be sure what is going on. Is this part of Emma's illness or her recovery? Is this a need she has, is it aggression, or both at the same time? Should I let her be, or challenge her? And *how* would I challenge her?

Bewildering as Emma's behaviour often is to me, I do not know whether this is an angry child testing my patience, needing to be stopped. Or is it a frightened teenager, trying to ward off what she most fears – nourishing herself, giving herself food. Am I being conned, used, abused or implored? Often, I do not know.

Emma will do this bottle-shaking many times over the next few weeks. Sometimes I walk away. Sometimes, sitting still beside her, I try to imagine what she might be going through and having to confront in her inner world.

Facing addiction, whether to food, drink or drugs, must be such a steep climb up, like a cliff wall. If she is to live, she must find her way to the top – to safety – using hand-holds, footholds on the way.

Perhaps I am a hand- or a foothold to Emma. Nothing personal. She is just using me to test the way, to climb up.

As her stay with me approaches Emma is heavy with terror. For, despite our talks and our time together, she knows how much she has hidden from me about her attitude to food and the consuming nature of her appetite.

We have spoken of many things, her relationship with Colleen, her fear of life, her childhood times with me, but as her weight has begun to rise she has not mentioned, any more, her fears about eating. Yet, at this time, she is still struggling with the choices between binge-eating and a return to starvation. Especially, she is struggling with whether to stay outside or to join with other people, accept their help, be part of the group.

Not knowing the extent of her ambivalence, I think it is the steep climb up which distresses her, not the lure of a slide back down. A terrible burden for her, therefore. How can she live with me, in my place, and hide the roaring lion inside her?

# Chapter Twenty-Two

## BRIGHTON

The years of Emma's life which should have involved her developing into womanhood have been given over to anorexia and spells in hospital. Because of this, she has come to feel safe in the Unit. With its quiet atmosphere, people around, but not intruding, mostly keeping to their rooms, there is an air of calmness about it, of order.

Coming to me, my home is also calm and orderly, but I belong so much in the outside world, hundreds of books, the guitar and papers on the desk. And, with me, she will miss being housed in a place which stays still, where people suffering from anorexia, their foibles, their needs and demands, are specially catered for and where she is not bedevilled by too much choice.

Many aspects of daily living are decided for her on the Unit: when to eat; how much to have; whether or not to have a walk; what time to go to bed. She dreads the comparative freedom of my flat:

> Tense, anxious, worried, scared – feelings about my weekend OUT THERE . . . i have next to no real idea of how to live my life without using food . . . it's always been there for me: my comfort, my love; my chosen weapon, my hate; my best friend in the whole entire world, the universe, because s/he never ever went away . . . Letting go, saying goodbye to this relationship is going to be excruciating.

While Emma is feeling this, I, on the other hand, am planning treats for us. I have suggested a day-trip to Brighton the weekend she comes out; a trip to the theatre; and a ballet she has asked me to book. Knowing it will be hard for both of us, and bracing myself for difficulties, I have worked on the premise that enjoyment in between the tough times is what we need.

Emma has other ideas:

> Worried that Carol may try to structure my time for me, as she has already done for Monday evening in buying tickets for us both to the theatre . . . there's enough rushing and struggling in my head and i can't handle any more without feeling unsafe to the point where i'm reaching out for my old friend yet again.

Yet Emma does not confide these fears about doing too much and, arriving on a sunny Friday evening to pick her up, the first sign of trouble is – she isn't there.

She is *somewhere*, a nurse tells me, a little anxiously, but not waiting for me in reception. Her belongings are near-by, though, clustered around a settee in the small common room: half a dozen carrier bags; a pot plant; some notebooks; painting books; and a small but heavy brown grip.

Checking the room which was Emma's until lunch-time today, its new occupant is a girl of Emma's age and, over the nurse's shoulder, I see her lying, lengthways, as I used to, fully clothed on top of the bed. She has long, sleek, dark hair, is around thirteen stone and looks as I have seen Emma do at this weight – full, lush.

There is a fairer girl sitting on the bed talking to her. Hair tied back in a bun, she is conferring with the dark girl in a gracious manner, a bit like an elder stateswoman, I realise, although she is the same age. This is Emma, as she is today, at her most frightened, her hair in a severe bun to make her look older, to make her believe she can cope.

Neither of them turns their head when the nurse comes in. Nor do they stop talking closely, quietly together when she says:

'Carol is here' – and then repeats it.

Still no response.

So, this is how it will be.

Five minutes later, while I am carrying some of her

belongings into the car, Emma emerges and, with her back to me, bends to pick up something from a chair.

'Hello,' I say with a smile, which she half responds to.

As we move the bags, Emma is increasingly tense and I notice the brown grip, which was heavy for me, she carries with ease, all seven stone of her.

On our way out over speed bumps in the road tomorrow's day-trip to Brighton is at the top of her list of immediate dreads: 'Is it going to interfere with my meal-plan?' she asks, in a strained voice.

'I have to eat at the times I'm supposed to.'

She goes over what these set times are: main meals at eight in the morning, noon, and five; with snacks in between at ten, three, and between eight and ten at night.

'There'll be cafés on the way, and we can take food with us as well if you like.'
Silence, but not the companionable kind.

At Emma's request, we stop, a short way off at a supermarket for the extra snacks she feels she must buy. Waiting in the car, it is a balmy, warm, summer's evening with blackbirds singing in the nearby trees and I am OK for at least fifteen minutes.

Then, a stab of anxiety. What if I have lost her? What if she doesn't come back, gets harmed while in my care? What if she just disappears?

I have never felt this way about her before, not as a child, when there was easy trust between us. She would always have come back, then. But now?

Forty minutes later, watching her walk towards me in that slow manner she has when she is at her most anxious, it is her way of slowing things down, I realise, of managing her terror. A way, too, of imposing her will. An army would not move her faster.

Back in the flat, trying to ease the tension, I say:

'Look, you don't have to come to Brighton if you don't want to. If that's what's bothering you, don't worry, I'll go on my own.

'You can have a day by yourself, laze around or read. Would you prefer that?'

Emma shakes her head: 'I'll come with you,' she says, her voice still strained.

And I leave it there. We have, in any case, had some luck. A neighbour who is away for a few days offers Emma her flat in the house next door. She can have a proper bed and some privacy. But as I take her in, watch how she is, I see it is not what she wants either.

She seems to need familiarity and the security of surroundings she knows and privacy at the same time. This goes for her thoughts about me as well. I think she wants me to be with her and for her to be allowed to ignore me when she wishes.

Emma *does* sleep next door, though, and the following morning she arrives at my place wearing only a skimpy black petticoat and briefs. Nothing else.

I look at her in surprise. She has walked from next door, along the front of two big houses on a through road

– and it is lightly raining too. I am flummoxed. Is this a wayward young woman walking a London street in her petticoat – or a child in her pyjamas wandering, innocently, next door?

'Aren't you cold?' I ask.

She shakes her head.

She is still very thin: white stick-like legs and arms; concave chest. With so little on, her body looks sad, forlorn, as if abandoned, and as if she is careless of being hurt, inviting it almost.

'What are you going to wear to Brighton?' I ask her.

'This,' she says.

'No,' I reply and, to my surprise, she accepts what I say. She needs to wear trousers, a cardigan, a coat and bring an umbrella, and – I round off with a smile – probably wellies too.

A good spell then, as we begin the journey. On the way through Elephant and Castle, Brixton, Streatham, we talk about clothes, music, and how she is managing with money (she is receiving disability benefit).

As we come towards Purley it is 11.20. Her meal due in forty minutes, I ask if she would like to hang around a while, find a café, be ready to eat when she is supposed to, or go on a bit and risk maybe being slightly out on the timing.

Emma choosing to go on, the road beyond Coulsdon seems, suddenly, restaurant-free, and as the fields and spaces of Surrey open out around us, it is my turn to feel tense.

Heading for the M23, my leg stiff on the accelerator pedal, there is tension all the way up my spine when, at last, a service station comes into view. Noon, exactly, as we drive into the forecourt.

Standing at the self-service counter, I find I am suddenly ravenous and, as Emma wanders off, nonchalantly, too nonchalantly I realise afterwards, to the loo, I set to. Gathering up a vast meal of gammon, egg, baked beans, chips, mushrooms, salt, vinegar, tomato sauce, more salt, more tomato sauce, I fall upon this plateful like a famished woman.

Coming back from what I later learn is a pre-lunch illicit snack in the loo, Emma messes her jacket potatoes and baked beans round and round the plate. Methodically, carefully almost, she pats, chops, squashes, pleats, forks over, digs, cuts, squashes, mashes, pleats, forks again until the whole lot is like anonymous mashed baby food which she eats slowly, chopping in between.

Just as well I have finished mine.

Setting off again, Emma asks if I am ever afraid of singing in the car, which is what I am doing.

'No,' I reply. 'Are you?'

She says she is. She is afraid people will look at her if she sings.

So I get her to sing along and, pretty soon, Brighton arrives and we have made it, sun shining and the sea glistening at us under a clear blue sky.

\*    \*    \*

On this day, as on others on our trips out, Emma's moods and her ages, her very person, change from one moment to the next: from joy to despair; from ease to tension; from eight years old to twenty or more.

With her first sight of the sea she is all these ages and full of joy. But half an hour later, walking out along the groynes at Rottingdean, I have lost her again. Surrounded by sun, breeze and glinting sea she is crying. Head down, shoulders slumped, she cannot take the beauty of it, she tells me. She wants to, wants to accept what is around her, but it hurts. All this life, all this sun, this sensation. It hurts her too much. She cannot stand it.

She spoils everything, she sobs. She is spoiling it for me now. She will never ever be happy, she will always spoil things.

Cradling her till she is calm again, I leave her for a while to walk along the path. But it is 2.45, almost her snack-time and, retracing my steps, she is there, where I left her, sitting on the beach. Head down, she is absorbed by now, like an old-fashioned child, picking up one stone, then another, turning it round, placing it back. Looking at pebbles. But she is nineteen, not nine.

Later, in and out of moods, I ask if she would like to see the Royal Pavilion and she looks rapturous at the sight of the dining room and the music room. Browsing around, late in the day by now, we end up in the gift and souvenir shop.

She slows again, insists on fingering things, looking at them, putting them down, picking up something near it, looking at it, putting it down, picking up the thing next to it. All with the studied slowness of someone who is willing her own time on the world.

The last customers there, I wait another minute or so before saying we must go, people want to shut up shop.

But she is in her own world and I am irritated. Anorexia's selfishness, its self-preoccupation, is something I find hard to accept and here is Emma at her most self-absorbed.

'I'll see you outside,' I say, and walk away.

Sitting outside in the sun I think of the clouds in her. One moment she is with me, the next the 'sun' in her withdrawn. She is such a weight at these times and, as so often with her illness, I cannot be sure when she is 'being ill' and being perverse.

It is shortly after six by the time she comes out, I ask if she would like to go home now, or stay by the sea a little longer.

She shrugs.

Walking back to the car, Brighton looks wonderful. Passing through a square, a hundred or more people are sitting at tables set out on the pavement, enjoying the evening air. It is good to hear voices, see people thronging, milling, laughing.

On the walk back along the front, a large man in his garden is stripped to the waist, lying down in full view of the street, beer in one hand, newspaper in the other, a smile on his face.

But Emma is behind her cloud.

# Chapter Twenty-Three

❧

## TENSE TIMES

The recovery plan Emma signs up to while she attends the Unit during the day involves having supervised meals in the company of other patients. Eating together in a proper dining area is seen as part of accepting food as a normal, social part of life, of demystifying it and bringing it out of the 'closet'.

It means, too, that staff can see how people are coping with the set meals they are prescribed. While there is no punishment for failing to eat the set amounts, privileges like phonecalls may be withdrawn if people fail to co-operate with the programme and they are, in any case, expected to talk about their problems with it. Thus, the private relationship a person has with food begins to be revealed and exposed to discussion, 'treatment' and recovery.

Central to the recovery programme, as well as eating in company, is the fact that patients stay with each other for

half an hour after the meal to let food digest, and to reduce
the chance of purging.

When she is on this programme as a day-patient, Emma
*seems*, on the surface, to be doing well but her diary reveals
otherwise:

> *Meal supervision has just ended and most of us are
> still seated in the lounge area . . . My body has
> tightened up, my breathing has quickened and i'm
> feeling tense and nervous . . . Fulfilling my appetite
> feels like giving in – anorexics don't <u>eat</u>, what on
> earth am i doing? . . .*
>
> *i can walk anorexia's tightrope whenever i choose,
> but i know that i can just as easily hide in the
> numb cocoon that is bulimia, or the lonely no-emotion
> of compulsive eating – these are my three playmates,
> and have been for as far back as my memory can
> stretch . . .*
>
> *They're not the best friends that a girl could
> have, but i've come to rely on them alone over 20
> years of my life. They've bruised me; scared me;
> burnt me; beaten me; buried me; sucked me dry of
> life. But they never left me. i learnt to rely on
> them, all my trust was fed into their bloodless veins
> because at least there, i know it would be safe.*

With this 'bloodlessness' deep inside her, Emma does not
feel comfortable at home with me. Nor I with her. She

is tense, prickly, hostile and I get the feeling she resents even my presence and wants me out of the way.

Often Emma does not seem to see or hear me and I start to feel unwelcome in my own home. Coming out of the study to fetch something, Emma, on the settee in the living room, will look at me as if I am disturbing her, which I am. In returning to secretly binge-eating, her (success-ful) efforts to conceal this from me create an awkward, difficult atmosphere.

Unaware as I am of this guilty secret of hers, Emma's anorexia seems even more tyrannical, alienating and ugly. I see how much she is physically changed, how much her expression changes when she is with her illness – and when she is with me.

The latter is affectionate, loving; the former is surly and aggressive, closing her down, making her blind to the outside world.

Deeply preoccupied in this mode, she thinks only of when I will stop talking, go out, or into the study so she can have her next bit of secreted-away, illicit, food.

This takes its toll on me. Friends are my refuge – and time. It will only be a few weeks, I tell myself, and the truth is I could not manage longer. I thank God for my sense in resisting pressure from Therese and limiting Emma's stay.

Emma's secret eating makes breakfast and her evening snack even more laboured and stressful.

There is the time when I have to close the study door while trying to work, and the living room door too, because of the loud noise coming from the kitchen – Emma's fierce chopping.

Her warm food sitting on a china plate, she is chop, chop, chopping it with a knife and fork, as if trying to kill it. She stops for a moment. Then the noise starts all over. Emma's relationship with her illness is a war zone again. Having made the decision to be on the food programme, I had thought outright hostilities would have ceased. But the demands of anorexia, and the way it takes over its host's territory, are not that easily assuaged:

*After all the years of running from myself, my fear/anger/desire/hate/emotion, i'm all of a sudden standing face to face with it all and there's nowhere to hide. I feel vulnerable and naked, and i want my eating disorder to rescue me so desperately . . .*

Turning to 'the enemy' for help in this way, Emma is torn between anorexia as friend and foe, as rescuer or saboteur. Which way will she turn – a step into the world, or a slide back into the familiarity of her illness?

She deflects this tension outwards and the battle between Emma's stated attempts at recovery, and her secret, forbidden eating, continues to affect the peace of my home.

As well as bottle-shakings, choppings and the ever-present conflict involved in Emma's food, there is the added tension of the craving which illicit eating has produced in her.

The latter makes of Emma someone she, herself, does not like: someone deceptive, sly, who, in the way of addicts, is so preoccupied with the next 'fix' that she will do anything to get it.

Appalled by the aggression in Emma, I am determined not to be a slave to her illness, which is what *it* – she – so easily demands.

The atmosphere of my flat so fundamentally disturbed, I become aware how much of my time Emma has consumed and of staff time at the Unit, too.

I see Emma and other patients treat staff as if they were servants sometimes. This is part of anorexia, I am told: its imperiousness, its demands and staff are able to take it.

I notice it one day at the Unit. While sitting waiting for a team meeting, a girl comes and sits opposite. Probably Emma's age, she is around six stone; grey; desperately ill-looking; distracted and, yes, ugly, because of the level of her self-involvement.

She paces, groans, puts her head in her hands, asks why the cab she is waiting for is so long in arriving, goes back to ask the nurse again and again.

Unable to sit still, disturbing the usually calm waiting area, her self-obsession, her dis-ease, seems to be all there is of her and when her eyes meet mine, they do not stay. In a sense, she cannot see me.

It is a lack of recognition I have come to understand through Emma, that there is something bigger than me, something, literally, more 'in her face'.

Emma's self-obsession is overwhelming during her stay with me and she would drag me into it if I let her. But I am determined not to collude. Talking to her, I sometimes try to by-pass her illness, ignore it if you like, for I can glimpse the girl behind it. And, when her illness is too much for me, I pull rank, speak to this girl, refuse, for a while, to engage in anything except ordinary practical matters: will we walk, or stay in?; will we watch TV together, or read?; will we have a chat, or an early night?

Perhaps surprisingly, Emma and I talk very little about her eating. She has not mentioned it after the early days when she was struggling with the choice of life or death, and I have not mentioned it either.

I think it would be too much for both of us for me to monitor her food as well. She already feels 'exposed' with me at times, and it seems an invasion of her privacy to step into this central 'place' which she so strongly guards. Considering how much of my 'interference' she has tolerated so far, part of her illness and her recovery must be hers, I believe, and nothing to do with me.

The aspect of Emma's illness I *can* help with is the other kind of food. Knowing her history, where she comes from, who she is without her illness, when she believes she is only a bad, worthless person I can sustain her with story-food from her past.

Even so, the going is rough. By the time our first weekend,

when we go to Brighton, is over, I am glad Emma is going away for the day – back to the Unit.

When she arrives at my place that morning from the flat next door she is tense and anxious. What will she feel about going back after a weekend away? she asks. What will she say to people on the Unit when they ask how her weekend went?

Kissing her goodbye, saying I will be here when she comes home, I tidy up from where she has left in a rush, gather up her laundry, then wash the stainless steel cups she uses to measure, precisely, the food she must eat. During the day, making the most of her time away, I settle to work.

But Emma does not come home to me that night, or any other night of this week. She comes in, yes, but barely says hello, and goes to the large dining table by the window where she has found another outlet for her obsession – a jigsaw.

Sitting there, in the evening sunshine, side on to me, she stays, for hours, saying nothing, not looking up, just doing the jigsaw. Rising when it is her snack-time, ignoring me as she passes to go to the kitchen, she then returns to the puzzle on the table.

Escaping to friends, I go out to eat, drink, chat, get away. But after three or four days, I have made a decision. Emma may need to hold on to some of her obsessive behaviour but not all of it.

There is the business of my going away soon. It is important she uses this time, learns to enjoy the flat, the lovely area I live in and not bury herself in cardboard pieces on the table.

Telling her this, saying I want her to use my time away to her advantage, I say she can do the jigsaw for a while, up to an hour. But no more.

She glares at me.

> Carol told me she doesn't want me to do as much of the puzzle . . . i know it's an avoidance mechanism, but i'm dealing with so much as it is — how dare she make me take on even more . . .
>
> There are so many aches and pains to struggle through, for the first time _ever_, i'm out unprotected in the middle of _being alive_. Without the filter of my eating disorder i'm experiencing the truth, the clarity, the harshness, the freshness of _being alive_ and it's absolutely terrifying. i want to curl up in a soft blanket and hide my body, my face, my self. i want to be unseen and unheard. Food is my voice. Food is the voice i use to speak to myself.

Emma is unable to take in, to ingest, any more when her illness fills her so much. Husky when she speaks to me, afraid to sing, anorexia is, indeed, in the middle of her.

So, we struggle, she and I, till I go to France. I think she will feel better without me, that she will find herself a little, experience some quiet and freedom, but she is ambivalent:

*Longing for oblivion . . . Anorexia and bulimia keep me so safe from those real pains* [of the world], *but open out into a whole other realm of (sur) real pains and aches . . . and death . . .*

*All i want to do is float quietly on my back, looking up at the blue sky and white clouds, until i can learn how to smile without drowning.*

# Chapter Twenty-Four

❦

# IF LOOKS COULD KILL

My trip to France is with the Alexander school I am train-ing at. We have been invited to join some other schools for a week near the French–German border in Alsace. Studying in the lovely woodland surroundings of a music academy, the food is tremendous, the weather great, and within hours of arriving on French soil, I forget Emma.

Wanting a clean break while away, I do not phone her. I have had enough of anorexia and am glad to be free of it.

Feeling light and unburdened I enjoy the beautiful surroundings and the work: the energy of dozens of people coming together and the buzz of human voices, high up in the hills.

We enjoy evening music, songs, entertainment, walks, wine-tasting, swimming, drives to local villages, the triptych in the museum at Colmar and the week quickly goes by.

It is not until the final day as we are driving back across France towards the ferry that thoughts of Emma return.

'You're quiet,' one of my passengers says and I find, as I have done with most of Emma's illness, that there is nothing I feel I can say. People close to me know what is going on, but, with others, I have no wish to repeat the complicated story of her illness.

A few miles from home, I feel even more anxious about what I may be coming back to. I would love to find nothing to contend with, but I cannot get my keys to work. They are part of a new set I had cut for Emma before leaving, but she found them stiff and difficult to use, so I had taken them to France with me, and given her mine instead. Now I cannot use them either. Tapping on the door, there is no responding movement or call from inside. Where is she?

Sitting on the staircase for a moment, I find my heart is pounding and I prepare myself for what I most dread – her death, her suicide. Most of the time I do not think of this, do not imagine it a likely prospect. Only when I am tired and stretched does this spectre of Emma's death trouble me.

But if it is there, it will have to be faced and, having another go, fumbling again in the hallway, at last I get the key to turn and go in.

Emma is not dead. She is sitting a few feet away at the head of the dining table, facing me, dressed all in black, with a snack in front of her where the jigsaw used to be. She does not move, stays sitting as she is, hands in her lap, the aloof lady of the house. She smiles at me, a controlled smile, and a controlled voice enquires of me, rather formally, whether I have had a nice time.

This begrudging acceptance of my return is recorded thus:

*i resent Carol for returning . . . i feel leaden and miserable. i want to have my own place. My week alone at Carol's proved to me that i can handle that.*

She had written a few days earlier she needed to tidy the flat – and had not got round to it. The place, as I enter, is messy, her stuff, like chickweed, invading the living room floor. It is the other kind of invasion which gets to me though, the human kind.

When Emma was visiting me as a sixteen-year-old, in the house where I lived a few years back, I had the impression there was something she wanted to claim – or even take – from me, and this seems to be it. Emma would like to live in my flat by herself without my annoying presence. Her need to possess is powerful and, by default, her wish for me to disappear.

Emma's wish for authority over me and mine would seem to be fuelled by the return of her own uncontrollable appetite. Although under eight stone at this time, she knows from past experience that when she begins to eat 'normally' again, as she has done for the last few months, her need for junk food kicks straight back in.

Like an addict, Emma had been bingeing while I was away, as she had been before I left, and as she plans to do on the nights when I go out to escape her:

*Carol will be out until 10.30pm. i could binge.*

Already I feel exhausted by her hostility. Avoiding her to begin with and then, eventually, trying to find some safe, uncontentious ground between us, I ask what she did while I was away.

She shrugs her shoulders.

Did she walk a little? I half suggest.

This produces a definite – adamant – response.

Emma did not walk while I was away she informs me, her voice rising, because her physiotherapist told her not to because that had been her obsession previously, to get physically over-excited and to do too much.

But surely a slow walk along the canal . . . ? I venture, and then realise my mistake.

When Emma is like this – angry, lying or, at best, exaggerating – I must not fall into her trap. She has always needed me to be outside it, different from other adults in her past, and I usually am. So I stop. Say no more.

But I am getting more and more rattled at feeling like an outsider in my own home, and by a week or so after my return, am determined this cannot go on. So far, Emma has returned from the Unit, sat listlessly in a chair, said nothing, and then we have both gone to bed.

What is the point of her being here? She has, after all, asked for my help with her illness, for she trusts me. It is implicit between us, this trust, as is the unspoken idea that I hold a key to her rescue: because I know her. I believe in her 'better self', in her ability for repair. I do not want to lose sight of this. But how to recover our closeness?

I decide we will do some housework. I could do it quickly on my own, but I want us to do something together. She had always enjoyed helping me in the past, and since we are off for another trip to the seaside on Saturday morning, Bournemouth this time, it would be nice if we were talking first.

I also suspect Emma has little idea what is involved in living in a place, that this is another one of those pieces of 'mother-food' she has not ingested. She is as unpossessed of the knowledge of how to care for a flat, as she is of herself. So, on Thursday morning, I say we will do some chores when she gets back from the Unit.

She is furious, absolutely not prepared for me to impose on her in this way:

'What do you mean, housework?' she almost shouts.

I say a bit of Hoovering, cleaning, things like that. Not very much.

Full of rage, she storms out.

That afternoon, in the middle of work, I get an unexpected

phonecall. Emma wants to know in detail what this house-work is going to consist of. Sounding as if we are negotiat-ing a contract, she asks for a precise account of what, exactly, I have in mind.

Surprised – and busy – I say not to worry, it will not be very much, and we will sort it out between us when she comes in.

But this will not do. As if reading from a legal docu-ment, Emma tells me she wants to know what will be expected of her, what tasks she will have to fulfil and how long they will take.

Irritated by this, I say I have work to do, cannot stay any longer, and will see her later.

Therese phones next. She says Emma has 'reported anx-iety' over the housework and that she is ringing to investigate.

As patiently as I can, I say it will not be onerous and that its main purpose is to benefit Emma. I believe she does not know how to do housework and that since she is soon to be living on her own, I could show her quickly and easily and she will probably be grateful.

'I think you'll find she doesn't know how to switch on a vacuum cleaner, or wash out a sink,' I say.

Therese is not satisfied. She says all this needs to be 'negotiated' with Emma.

At which point, I lose patience:

'Look, I've known her since childhood. She knows she can trust me. Now I have work to get on with.'

The argument which takes place that evening is short

and to the point. Returning home late, Emma looks furious, as she did in the morning, and does not return my
'hello' from where I am ironing in the kitchen.

Instead she tells me, straight out, that I have no right whatever to organise her life for her. She had things planned
for this evening and she is extremely angry that I have
interfered.

I say that while she is living in my place I expect her
to treat me and my home with respect, which involves
helping out a little. I have, after all, washed and ironed for
her since she has been here.

'You offered,' she says scornfully – and I am quick to
respond, letting her know she does herself no favours by
despising my, or anyone else's, kindness.

I tell her, too, that the housework is for her benefit, for
when she has a place of her own. Keeping a place clean
and enjoyable to live in need not be difficult if she knows
how.

Hearing this, softening, Emma agrees it will be a good
thing and, slowly, we move towards working together, to
being in accord for the first time since she has stayed with
me.

Her remaining anger taken out on the scourer, the sink
is spanking clean within five minutes, rinsed out, and shining, and she is smiling. What's next? she wants to know.

Having a tea-break, she asks about what kind of cleaner she should buy. Can she get those sink scourers in any
supermarket? How long should you use a dishcloth for?

Running her hand along the smooth surface she has just worked on, Emma is delighted:

'I'm enjoying this! And I'm so looking forward to doing it in a flat of my own.'

## Chapter Twenty-Five

*❦*

# BOURNEMOUTH, VIENNA AND LIFE

In the good patches between us, when she is calm and receptive, Emma and I deal with the gaps in her everyday knowledge of how to live a life: how to take care of herself; and how to use systems – like registering to belong to a library, for example. She is embarrassed to ask most people – and she and I do what we can.

She is frustrated from not knowing how the world works, or to get it to work for her, and this easily drives her to be angry or withdrawn.

Walking with her to the hole-in-the-wall one sunny evening to withdraw some cash for her snacks, she is at a loss about how much to take out, for she has seldom handled money. Most of the disability benefit which supports her is still in the bank. She has no real idea what things cost and how often she should withdraw money or how much she should carry with her.

So I suggest £20–£30 and sit on some steps to enjoy the late afternoon sun while she goes to the cash dispenser.

She is back in a minute and furious. The machine has eaten her card, and she looks as if the world has come to an end. Going to the screen with her to see what it shows, she is sharp: 'What are you looking for?' she demands. 'I told you what it said.'

In our good times together when she is able to take things in, I do as much filling in and filling up as I can, and talk about where this seeming inadequacy of hers comes from. The world is not against her, I say. Nor is she stupid, as she often calls herself. It is just that, when she was a child, she turned her back on key bits of information.

'You're still young enough to ask,' I say, giving her a hug. 'Soon you won't be. So, ask away.'

Sometimes, though, I am weary of the extent of Emma's unpossession – as with events when we go to Bournemouth. We are lucky with the weather as we drive to the sea. The journey is sunny, Emma companionable, and we look set for a fair time.

Finding two single rooms in a hotel near the front, after an hour or two's walk, it is getting near to dinner time, and we both need food. Testing herself, I realise, doing as I have suggested, Emma asks if she can pick the restaurant.

'Fine,' I say.

Walking down a street with eateries along practically the whole length, both sides, forty minutes later we are both still hungry. Emma is discovering the bewilderment of too much choice. Almost frozen with weighing up one against the other, she asks if I would like to choose and I say the good-quality Chinese would do for me, but she is vegetarian and has said their veggie dishes are not up to scratch for her.

Almost an hour later, we are in the worst restaurant in Bournemouth. It has a dark interior, loud music, jokey signs and ominous street theatre. Looking through the window, I see three bouncers in the pub over the road strut their stuff, flexing muscles for the night's work ahead.

Things do not improve.

Emma takes an age choosing between a veggieburger and potato skins in cheese with coleslaw as a side dish. She is nervous and asks incessant questions: what is in the cocktails; what do they taste like; how big is four ounces; do they have sweet wine?

Then she is worried the burger might be too big or too small. This is not how I like to eat.

After the meal, Emma is distraught. Initially saying she is not up for an after-dinner walk, and will go back to the hotel, she then says she has eaten too much, and wants to be sick.

So, we walk, slowly, until she calms a little. Thinking, after a while, she will probably be all right, we both turn in early, at around nine.

By 9.30 *I* am desperate: noisy celebrations and loud music from a wedding party in a downstairs room of the hotel. I have a friend in Bournemouth, Sheila, and, knocking on Emma's door, I ask if she would be OK if I went out for an hour.

Emma, I realise later, is in euphoric mood. Through the crack in her door she gaily tells me that of course she doesn't mind me going out. She will be fine.

But she isn't. She was bingeing, as she tells me, years later, and hurriedly hiding food as she heard my call from the corridor. When she buys the chocolate bars, crisps and biscuits I do not know, nor where she hides them, but as I go out that night to escape from her, she settles down to eat.

Sheila has nieces of Emma's age and is a good listener. By the time I return to the hotel an hour later, I am ready to sleep through a dozen wedding parties.

Off to the headland the next day: Hengistbury Head, sea all round, marvellous views, birds in the shrubs – and a storm. The sky above is fine, but Emma is suddenly distraught again, beset by terror.

I have not explained enough to her where we are going, what we are doing, how long it will take, when we will be back and, startled by this place seeming wild and far away from anywhere, it is too much for her.

She is never going to be well, she tells me, sobbing. She feels like a five-year-old but is angry with me for treating her like a child. And then she feels nineteen, and she feels all these different ages at the same time, and it means she doesn't know who she is, and doesn't know what to do, and it will never, ever, be all right.

Holding her I am torn between exasperation at the patience Emma's illness demands, and the wish to soothe her. I wonder if she will ever be well and if I will have enough reserves to continue.

On the journey home she sleeps all the way. Glancing at her, seeing how ill she looks, and how genuinely exhausted, I know I must help as best I can. But will it be enough?

For me, perhaps for both of us, there is rescue at hand with a trip to Vienna a short while after, for a copyright conference I have to attend. I am glad to leave home and Emma will have left my place to stay in a hostel by the time I return.

Packing for four days away, I decide, as an afterthought, to put in a recently acquired green frock – just in case. Shot silk, off the shoulder, mid-calf, it is a dance frock, a dinner frock – a proper frock.

'Do you have a lifestyle to support this?' the shop assistant had asked in friendly manner when I bought it.

'No,' I had said. 'But I intend to get one.'

So, Vienna, home of string quartets, Viennese waltzes and, at this time, the Austrian presidency too. Perhaps the end-of-conference dinner would be held somewhere special, somewhere where a jade green frock and dancing shoes would not be out of place.

And, after the last speech closes, an announcement is made: that dinner will be held in a palace near-by. Usually closed for the summer, it will be opened especially for the occasion.

It is just as a palace should be, beautiful, like something from a fairy tale: murals; paintings; and an oval ballroom with floor-length windows leading out onto balconies overlooking the gardens. And, indeed, there is a quartet playing Viennese waltzes, and as dancing begins, the frock truly comes into its own, swirling round and round – me inside.

'I'm getting dizzy,' I gasp at the chest of the tall, dinner-suited stranger who has me in his arms. 'We'll have to stop.'

'Just hold on to me,' he commands.

And I do.

Returning to London, my home is calm, peaceful and has been cared for and tidied before Emma left. I am glad. Thinking about her while away, I have wondered how she would cope with the move, and how she would be feeling. Enjoying getting dressed for the dance, looking in the mirror, I had longed for the time when Emma might do the same, wished, as I have barely dared to, for her to find her own happy reflection in the glass.

A few hours later, I find her card propped on a cupboard:

*Thank you Carol, for letting me share your home with you over the last few weeks. i know that it's been a huge strain on you, and so i want you to know just how much i've appreciated your love and support, without which i'd have been completely lost. i feel that i've learnt a great deal about how to live life well and efficiently from you, which i've* needed for a long time, and now value very much – (with the exception of 'that' [the housework] argument which was _far_ too horrible for words and made me feel about five years old!!! But it would have been much _much_ worse if it was with anyone other than you).

   i love you very much.

   Emma.

# Chapter Twenty-Six

≈§

## SURVIVING THE SMOKE ZONE

After returning from Vienna, Emma having moved to sleep in a hostel, still attending the Unit by day, I notice things missing, sweet stuffs mainly: most of the top off a rhubarb crumble; and a bag of brown sugar nearly gone. I wonder whether to say anything when Emma and I meet to go to the ballet, but by the time the evening has arrived, I have forgotten.

Instead I remark how nice she looks in a simple black mini-dress with a low-slung belt and a black cardigan. Around eight stone at this time, Emma looks slender and well and, as we sit on the bus heading towards central London on a sultry summer's evening, tells me what she has been doing.

She went to a party, she says, with people she had kept in touch with from her A-level course. She was nervous about going, about what to say and how to behave, but decided she would 'be herself' and listen to other people when she felt nervous.

But everyone was doing something, she noticed, and had something to talk *about*. Most of them were in university and chatted about their courses, activities and new friends. Others had jobs and talked about work and colleagues. She thought she was probably the only person who wasn't doing anything, who had nothing interesting to say.

She met a boy, though, about her age, and she would like to ring him. Is it all right to do that, she wants to know, and what will happen if he tells her to get lost? She would be devastated.

Happy to be listening to her, hearing her talk so openly, I know how much I would miss Emma if she were not in my life. But the next couple of months will be extraordinarily difficult, me torn between affection for Emma and the need not to be pulled under as problem after wearying problem emerges.

There is the hostel where she is staying, for example, until the so-far elusive flat is found for her to live in permanently. While reassuringly small and homely – only six people in a specially converted house, each with their own room, and a communal kitchen and living room – every one of the other five 'inmates' as Emma takes to calling them, smokes. She is distraught by this, and afraid to say anything at the Unit because 'they' have put her there.

She feels oppressed and invaded, and since smoking is prohibited in individuals' rooms, it takes place in the communal lounge, which is next to Emma's bedroom and lies between it and the kitchen. In order to avoid walking through the smoke zone, she begins stacking up dirty supper dishes and laundry in the small space she lives in.

Knowing there is only so much chaos she can take, and fearing where it will end up, at Emma's request I phone Therese to ask how the flat-search is going. She says what I know to be true – that Emma is lucky to have anywhere at all and that she has other people to think about. She is doing what she can and Emma will have to wait.

At the hostel, Emma is also upset that the staff and helpers on duty are young and inexperienced. She says she wouldn't feel confident to rely on them or to ask for emotional support. I think she is right. Meeting the young woman assigned to Emma's case when she eventually moves into her flat, it is Emma who ends up listening to the helper's problems.

At the Unit, things are difficult too. Emma tells me that Sonia, the dietician whom she used to see once a week, now says once every three weeks is enough. Emma says she doesn't think it is. She wants more, but Sonia is clear about her decision. In her professional opinion, Emma can manage.

This is followed by someone forgetting to put in Emma's menus for the week, so she gets no food brought up at meal-times. She is upset, feels abandoned, and thinks of not eating again. Instead, she goes down to the kitchen to fetch a meal for herself – which is what she does all week.

Then, she says, the nurses on the Unit are not asking about her eating any more. She confesses she has been bingeing, and it was only a chance question by someone which got this information out of her.

'They think you're getting better,' I say.

But Emma is adamant about something. As she wants her illness her own way, so it is with her recovery. She wants it her way, in her time, at her pace. She wants to be the person who walks away from the Unit and from her illness. She does not want to be 'shoved out'.

We agree I will ring Therese to get some clearer guide-lines about what Emma should expect on the Unit at this time. Maybe, as a day-patient, it is normal for nurses not to ask about her eating. If this is the case, she agrees she would feel better about it. For her part, Emma will drop Sonia a note saying she is afraid of back-sliding and thinks she needs more support, so please could they talk about it some more.

It goes on in this way, with a new crisis every day or so for me to help unravel, practical and emotional problems entwined: a lost or misplaced travel card; whether or not Emma is ready to see her mother again yet, for she has not seen Colleen for four months; where she should buy new underwear; what kind to choose.

When Emma phones with these problems, I deal with them by being practical where possible and getting Emma to do her bit – what I think she can, and should, manage. I find it hard not to feel swamped. Unlike therapists or doctors, I do not have the ability to switch off and I carry her difficulties with me.

We both look forward to her leaving the hostel for a place of her own. But as the weeks go by, and it is summertime, with people on holidays, the bureaucratic machinery slows down.

Therese is ill, with no replacement. Just a caseload, with Emma in it somewhere, piling up on her desk. Emma's therapist is on holiday. Staff from the Unit are away too and, in the bleak evening times at the hostel, smoke all around her, Emma is lost.

Going for a break myself – a long weekend visiting friends in Scotland – I phone Emma a couple of times to make sure she is managing. She is not.

On the Sunday I am away she locks herself out of her room at the hostel, leaves the key at a friend's, who will be out for the evening, and has to wait for a master key to be fetched. A part of me wonders if she did this deliberately. Sitting in the park, until 10 p.m., not prepared to come back into the commonroom where the smoke is, she feels as if she is going to break apart. Rocking back and forth, keening, she is beset by wave upon wave of panic.

Surviving this, getting to her bed at last, the following day she is told a flat which looked a likely prospect has fallen through. The search for another one is on, but it is now late August and it will be early October, probably, before a place can be found.

I can see how wearing it must be for the people who

do the job of finding a place for Emma. Working on her behalf, often in under-staffed places with many 'Emma's' on their list – people who lose their keys on a regular basis, getting staff out at the weekend to let them in. But I am on Emma's side.

Meanwhile there is some good news. I have booked for us to go to Crete in late September, something I had promised Emma while she was an in-patient, a trip to a Greek island. Emma is delighted and so am I. I have not been to Crete for years and look forward to returning. I look forward to Emma enjoying herself, too. She is a strong swimmer and will spend lots of time in the water, I hope. She is hunched over still, her shoulders rounded and stooped and it may build her confidence and physical strength.

But, over the next few weeks, it gets even tougher. Emma is depressed and there are phonecalls from her most days, all of which I find exhausting. She is at the point of possible relapse, she says.

Has she told anyone on the Unit? I ask.

Silence.

'Emma, you must tell a nurse, or a doctor.'

Still she says nothing.

'Do you want me to do it for you?'

Then Emma's husky, strangled voice: 'No, I'll do it.'

'I'd like to know what they say. Will you ring me afterwards and tell me?'

But by 'afterwards' there is another crisis. Now that her weight is rising, her period has started back. She cannot cope at all. This is the time when she relapsed before.

'You must tell a nurse,' I say.

'The world is terrifying me,' she cries.

'Even knowing I'm dying isn't nearly as frightening as this.'

And for my part, I am exhausted. Friends are *my* support and talking to Ann, someone I have known for many years, she warns me to try and keep more distance.

'There must be more than one therapist there,' she says. 'They must have systems to cope with things like this. People relapsing is part of their work.

'And I wouldn't call Crete a holiday if I were you,' she warns. 'It may be for Emma, but don't count this as your time off.'

Wise words, as it turns out. But before Emma and I go to Crete, there will be one more 'event', one more important meeting which will help me understand the depth of Emma's fear that an independent life is something she will never be able to grasp hold of, or maintain.

The following week, I meet her father.

# Chapter Twenty-Seven

~§

## EMMA'S FATHER . . .

Emma's father makes major appearances in her diaries at certain times. At others he is absent. After leaving the family when Emma was a toddler, he re-emerged when she was around five and, soon after, began writing to her and travelling from Ireland to visit around half a dozen times a year.

Emma found these get-togethers distressing and, as she recalls, they disrupted her life. She barely knew her father and his behaviour towards her was, therefore, even more odd. Not seeming to realise she was a child he spoke to her as if she was a captive adult audience: details of the dangers, the frustrations, the inadequacies of the world and, obliquely, of his own life.

While she sat, barely saying a word, he talked of events she was not capable of understanding: about people she had not met; about newspaper headlines and TV reports;

about politics and injustices, road accidents and bad travelling conditions. All of which she found alien and, eventually, terrifying because she was unable to find her part in what was being said.

While he did her no physical harm, emotionally the damaging effect was substantial. He held a strange view of her, as some kind of cypher, and was not interested in her life: what she did; how she played; her schoolfriends; her child's days.

Instead, by the time she was eight or nine, he demanded she reply to his letters, containing, as they did, adult information about an adult world and about people in his personal life she had never heard of. If she did not do this and did not pay attention to the detail of what he wrote she was scolded in his next letter, or when he next saw her, for being a bad, ungrateful child.

Whatever it was her father wanted, Emma did not know how to provide it. She felt confused by what he did, and imagined the problem was a lack in her, rather than him. And there was something else:

*My dad was always late when we had our meetings – i never wanted to go in the first place, and then i'd be sitting and waiting, feeling so ugly and worthless because i wasn't worth being on time for . . . One time when my father was late he said he fell asleep . . . I wouldn't let myself cry in front of him.*

At the time she writes these entries about her father she reveals that she is also grappling with her feelings about sex, trying to understand why she is both attracted and repelled by the thought of it:

> I don't want to admit that one of my body's needs, and one of my emotional needs, is for sex . . . maybe it's the feeling of being used that frightens me so much . . . i don't want to be the one giving everything . . . I do want to love, and to <u>be</u> loved – I just don't want to feel how my father made me feel . . . I don't want to feel like the target for my father's expression of <u>his</u> insecurities/anger/ selfishness.

In making strong connections between what happened to her in the past and how she feels in the present, Emma writes of how her unrewarding relationship with her father affected her wish to grow up and have relationships.

Her negative view of men, and her way of trying to shut them out, relates directly to her anger towards her father. As she delves deeper, the entries fluctuate between hatred, anxiety and a need to love the man who has always let her down:

> I want to open myself out to a man's love, not a man's hate – i need to unlearn what my father taught me, i need to confront him and tell him how much

*hatred i have inside of me as a result of what he did . . . I want to have an adult conversation with him, explaining to him my understanding of my life and his part in it . . .*

*I want my dad to hug me and love me . . . I want him to be a part of my life. I want to know all about him and know why he is the way he is. I want to be able to love him or at least find some bits of him that aren't so negative . . . I wish i could hate him. But he's my daddy and i want him back.*

As she gets older, and continues to see her father on his occasional visits to London, Emma becomes angrier with him. She writes of the long-term harm to her in relating to a man who, as she tells it, denied her childhood and was blind to her identity:

*You obliterate my central sun and i hate and fear you for it . . . every moment with you is fraught with my anxiety of failure to be who you want me to be, to say what you want me to say . . .*

*You don't remember you have a daughter. You never see my pain. You see yourself.*

There was another problem with Emma's father, difficult for a small child who already thought of herself as greedy – his way of trying to keep her attention, to bribe her, with gifts. On each of his visits he would appear with presents, beautifully wrapped. And her confusion that she liked – and wanted – the presents, but not the man, was painful. He used 'sparkly Sellotape' and cut things into nice shapes and she wistfully writes:

*I wish he'd been able to translate that care into his treatment of me.*

Meeting him in the summer of 1998, combined with reading her diary entries, makes me understand more fully the size of the obstacles Emma faced as a child. Trying to find her way in the world, to find the vein of optimism, the intrinsic acceptance usually present in children, that her needs for growth, for nourishment, for recognition, would be met, she failed.

Instead of growing in ease and confidence, she was the somewhat anxious child I have memories of: unadventurous; hanging back; afraid of trying and of asking. A picture I carry in my mind of Emma's fear and reticence comes from when she was around eight or nine. Bringing her home for a big one, a long two-night stay. It was wintertime, and, for me, the end of an especially hard week.

Explaining to Emma that I needed to have a rest before we played some music, we both curled up on the floor. Lying next to the fire to read, Emma near-by, I, like her father, fell asleep. I remember nothing more till waking up

with her sitting close, looking down at me, her body tense
with worry:

'Are you all right, Carol?'

'I'm fine,' I say, slowly coming to, 'but have you been on
your own for a long time?'

A sad – a really sad – nod of her head.

'Well, why didn't you wake me?'

'I didn't like to.'

# Chapter Twenty-Eight

❦

## . . . AND MEETING HIM

Experts tell us that people who suffer from anorexia become ill when they do – usually around puberty – in an attempt to remain children and avoid growing into full sexual beings. Often, in girls, the desire not to become a woman involves a determined wish not to 'repeat' the mother – to grow up like her. It can also involve a corresponding wish to avoid male attention. In a poem, first written in 1997, Emma writes of her relationship with her father:

> Father/daughter
> Half/quarter
> split them apart
> break them apart
> stamp on them hard
> until they shatter

> *beat them hard*
> *until they don't matter*
> *and he can never hurt me again.*

At around the time I go with her to meet him in the summer of 1998, the poem is repeated, with just one difference, the underlining of the word 'never.'

Since her eighteenth birthday Emma's father no longer has visiting rights, and she has not seen him since she has been ill on this last loop of anorexia. She had written a few years back, to say she was very poorly in hospital, and had received no reply. Now, he has written to say he will be in London and wishes to see her one afternoon when she and I have planned to shop for Emma's 'new-look' wardrobe.

The letter has clearly upset her and she tells me she doesn't want to see him. She says it is because he gets angry at her, 'at the slightest little thing' and then she clams up and he gets even angrier: 'It feels like he's attacking me all the time.'

I suggest coming with her to meet him – at least for a coffee. She can tell him she and I are going shopping, and that we will join him afterwards.

'I'll be on your side,' I say.

Emma is happier then, for it seems she has imagined, strangely, I might be on *his* side. The sense of helplessness he produces in her makes her lose perspective.

'I don't think anyone has ever wanted to see it from my point of view before,' she says.

'I'd go home crying after I'd seen him and my mother would use it as a chance to air her grievances about him. She'd say things like:

'"That's why I left him. He was always like that," and she'd talk about herself and not me.'

We agree a meeting place for the three of us on the following Thursday, outside a shop in Tottenham Court Road.

That day Emma turns up looking awful: pale; stooped over; arms hanging by her sides, and she is wearing shiny black nylon trousers, a skimpy black corded top and big platform shoes.

In a department store I head for the jackets. She tries one on, simply cut in grey and dark brown weave, and stands there, shoulders stopped, stomach pressed forward, head down. She isn't giving the jacket a chance, I tell her. It needs a person inside it, not a conscript.

So, on to the next. This one is lighter and the collar curved rather than straight-edged, which suits her better. It has a grey-green weave, and looks lovely. At last she smiles, comes alive. Yes, this one looks good. She can see it for herself.

We do not buy one yet. Emma is not ready, so this excursion is a test run. She does, however, buy a sarong to wear on the beach in Crete.

Arriving slightly early for the meeting with her father, we lean against a wall across the road from the shop, chatting initially, until, head down again, she falls silent. I ask what's wrong.

She is afraid of him, she says, frightened of him flying into a rage 'at the tiniest thing'.

'Even if I look the other way when he's talking to me, if I do the tiniest thing wrong. I have to be perfect.'

A few minutes later, I spot him from across the busy street – or at least imagine I do. How can I know, for I have never seen a photograph of him, or been told what he looks like. But it *is* him. He is around forty-five to fifty, with dark greying hair and blue eyes, is tall, thin and stooped, and walks with a nervous tilt. More than anything, from this distance, he appears agitated and lost.

Emma goes to fetch him. As they stand, apart from each other, Emma looking distressed and lost, he becomes more and more agitated. Speaking fast, at Emma sometimes, but mostly to the world at large, his words run into each other and I find it difficult to catch what he is saying. Emma is silent, gazing at him, as he continues talking.

None of this is 'normal' and, distressed for Emma, wanting to protect her, I try and stop it, interrupt the tirade.

'I'm Carol,' I say, trying to gain his attention.

He ignores me, but Emma says something at last:

'This is Carol. She's been visiting me in hospital.'

Having to look at me, briefly, but obviously vexed by my presence, and unable to conceal it, his face is like that of a fifty-year-old child. It is the strongest impression I have of him, that of a fretful child, unable to stay still enough to take in his surroundings.

Trying to keep his attention, to calm him down, I ask ordinary things about how long he is in London and if he is enjoying his visit. He can barely wait till I have finished speaking before turning to Emma.

I watch them both as he takes her off into the shop, me following behind. Behaving as if he is showing a little girl around, wandering from counter to counter, picking up things, he points them out to her again and again, talking all the while as he goes on, from place to place, object to object.

Obsessively.

She is required to say nothing but look where he points, then back to him, then to where he points again. I am almost in tears at her misery, how mute she is, how still, how pencilled out and not herself she has become, her face like a blank page.

I cannot bear to watch, to see both their pain, Emma's exhausted face and his lost one. Approaching Emma, taking her aside for a moment for a long goodbye hug, I whisper I will be at home waiting for her to phone me later and not to worry, we'll sort things out.

Calling the following day, Emma says she could not ring sooner because she was with her father till after midnight. They went to a film. He talked, and talked. She says she felt bad, depressed and exhausted when she got back to the hostel.

I ask why she hadn't left, said she was tired, unwell.

'I still have a child-like terror of him,' she tells me. 'That if I don't do as he wants, be as he wants, he's going to come and get me. I'm really frightened of him.'

Then, in a stronger tone of voice, she says:

'In the shop with me, he obviously thought he was responsible, but it was me who was being responsible, but I couldn't tell him that.

'I felt so unsafe with him. It was such a struggle for me to keep us both going. It was unnatural and he didn't have a clue.

'I couldn't eat anything all the time I was with him.'

She has eaten today, thank heavens, but since she is seeing her father again, she is still vulnerable. I try and explain that what her father does is not necessarily his fault, but it is not the way most fathers behave with their daughters.

Changing tack, she asks if she should go to her dance class tomorrow, the Absolute Beginners class, which we had discussed she join up for. I say yes, and not to mind making a fool of herself and being awkward or anything. Because we have all done it more than once. She laughs, and I long for the time when I hear more of this laughter.

As Emma's father leaves, there is good news on the housing front, a possible flat. While it will not be empty until after we come back from Crete, and will need decorating and recarpeting, if she likes it, it will be hers to move into after we return. Excitedly, she rings to ask if I will come to see it with her and attend a meeting at the Unit to discuss it.

Of course I will. How lovely to hear the lift in her voice, and how optimistic she sounds. What a marvellous prospect, a home for Emma at last.

# Chapter Twenty-Nine

⋰∾

## THE KNOCK

The meeting at the Unit preceding us viewing Emma's flat
is problematic. I am puzzled by why they have done it this
way – meeting *before* she sees the flat – but it becomes
clear.

Housing in London being so difficult to arrange, she is
being told this is the flat, whether she likes it or not. If
she refuses to move in, she will be faced with a long wait
and even more time spent at the hostel.

Or else she will be moved somewhere further away, on
the outskirts of London, where accommodation is easier
to find, but where she would not be near her friends.

There are only a few people present at this meeting:
Therese; a young, dark-haired doctor I have not met before;
Emma's new therapist; a nurse and a medical student. It
begins with the doctor asking Emma how she is and she
says nothing. Just clams up.

I glance at her, surprised, and, her voice badly strained, she eventually says:

'Well, I'm a lot better than I was at the beginning of the year . . .'

The doctor who is chairing the meeting accepts this at face value. Nodding enthusiastically, he says, yes, she has made progress and is ready to take the next step towards recovery – a place of her own. He is sure she will like the flat which has been found for her. And that is that. No more said, the meeting set to end less than five minutes in.

Emma looks anxious and withdrawn. She has not seen the flat yet, and had imagined she would be told about it and have some things explained to her. There are all kinds of questions she wants to ask, about redecoration, for example. Will she be able to choose colours for it herself, and what about curtains? Is there a garden? Is she allowed to change things in it?

Knowing how anxious she must be feeling, and perhaps trapped, too, by the fact that acceptance is more or less being forced on her, I ask if it is possible to do anything about 'the knock'.

Emma has been told it is compulsory, a daily knock on her door by Dawn, a helper from Care in the Community. Living in what is classified as semi-sheltered accommodation, she will be free to live her life, but be kept an eye on as well to make sure she is all right.

Dawn will also be checking to make sure Emma is

looking after the flat. It makes sense. I can see why it has to happen and how there would be complaints and possibly tragedies if vulnerable young people were not checked up on.

But Emma feels overwhelmed by Dawn. Around Emma's age, she talks a lot, pouring out her problems, and leaves Emma feeling depressed and exhausted.

Emma doesn't want to be seen to be awkward. Nor does she want to get Dawn into trouble, but she asks me if there is a way round 'the knock', if she could see as little of her helper as possible. I have suggested a phonecall instead. Emma's responsibility, then, to be there to receive it.

The meeting is silent, again. Awkward. Then Emma's new therapist speaks up, says she and Emma should discuss this and see what might be achieved. But the doctor, who has been getting impatient, is not happy. It is compulsory, he says, the knock, and he puts in a new twist, saying that if Emma decides to reject the flat and goes for private accommodation instead, nasty landlords could come into her flat whenever they liked.

The rest of us are astonished, and Therese interjects:

'That's not right. They have to make appointments . . .'

But he continues. They don't make appointments, he says: 'I've had experience of it. They just come in.'

And that is that.

On the way out of the Unit, I tell Emma what the doctor has said is decidedly 'iffy'. Does she know him?

She shakes her head.

Outside, in the open, she introduces me to a friend of hers, who looks healthy, thank God, but we are outdoors, ready to go and see the flat, and Emma's friend is wearing a pale blue satin petticoat, or short nightie, with a black cardigan on top. I think maybe they come out into the grounds in their nightwear. But no, in typical anorexic style they have read the fashion magazines literally. This is their version of thin girls in strappy clothes.

The girl in the petticoat talks to me, as Emma has done on occasion, in a rather grand style, as if she is a 'lady' of some substance and I a visiting guest.

Do they chat much about clothes? I ask Emma in the car.

She shakes her head.

So, does she, Emma, see the difference between underwear or nightwear and 'going out' clothes?

'Yes,' she says, her voice strained again. 'But it's one of the things you don't know properly when you're ill and confused. You see these pictures and the people in the magazines are real for you.'

On the drive to the flat, in a north London suburb, fervently hoping it will be pleasant, I sense Emma's tension again. She knows it will be difficult for her to refuse it. We could do a lot of course to make it homely, brighten it up.

But we are both pleasantly surprised. It is one of two in a red-brick semi, Emma with the bottom half and two people sharing a similar flat on top. It has a good-size bedroom and living room, and a kitchen-diner with a bathroom leading off it.

It also has a garden with a clothes line. Emma grins broadly. After living in the hostel, it is one of the things she has most looked forward to – hanging her clothes out to dry in the fresh air, pressing them against her face, smelling the cleanness.

Her helper, Dawn, is there, and we look at what is needed to make it ready to move into. It will take a few weeks, perhaps, but should be ready by the time we come back from Crete.

On the way back to the Unit, Emma pleased with the flat, I imagine life is opening out for her. But after a while, Emma talks of fears about her parents. The Unit wants her to have family therapy, with her father, and with Colleen and Paul.

She is frightened because she feels neither of her parents knows who she is, and that faced with them, she will curl up, withdraw, say nothing and, possibly, relapse. For she still wants Colleen to know how much she is hurting and, faced with her mother, Emma is fearful she might go back into self-harm.

She is not ready for a meeting of this kind, she says. Part of her still wants her mother to take notice of her pain, to say to Colleen: 'Look, I'm dying.'

So, while there is a home in prospect, a place of her own at last, Emma's inner home remains under siege. Feelings of hurt, need, anger still consume her.

In the next few weeks, as we head towards our holiday, there are many anxious calls from Emma: about the progress of the flat; how much money to bring on holiday; what to wear; what the temperature will be like, etc.

The seemingly good news she can move into her flat before we go away has the effect of unsettling her. Emma thinks and moves slowly, and needs to 'fix' things, to control them in order to feel safe, for anything new and unexpected causes her alarm.

And there are other problems with the move, due mainly to lack of communication: people not turning up to switch on the gas; keys not available; a back door that doesn't lock; no new carpet fitted; decorating not finished; noisy people upstairs. Her diary, a few days before we fly, reveals she is exhausted and binge-eating:

> *I threw up dinner, then ate all the groceries I bought to last me over the weekend, then threw them up too . . . the thought of packing for Crete is feeling like an impossible task. I have a cold too.*

At my place, a few days later, sleeping over to catch an early morning flight from Gatwick, she records bingeing in the middle of the night:

*1 banana + fruit and nut bar + yogurt flapjack (eaten secretly in the dark in Carol's living room half hidden under the covers).*

# Chapter Thirty

୬ଽ

## CRETE

Arriving at my place on the eve of our trip to Crete, Emma has visibly gained weight in the couple of weeks since I have last seen her, from eight and a half to nine stone, and I am glad to see her looking so well. As she comes in, I give her a hug, say how good she is looking and she bursts into tears.

Saying she is fed up with people commenting on how she looks, only Emma knows what she is doing under wraps, in the dark, and how dangerous her bingeing is. At this rate, she could be back in a loop, heading towards fourteen stone by Christmas.

I, however, am in the dark again and imagine her outburst is another 'teenage tantrum', Emma arriving as her fifteen-year-old self rather than the woman who has just had her twentieth birthday.

But her first sights of Crete, of the sky, the sea, the

mountains, and the village of Palaiochora, where we are staying, thrills her. As we sit on a bus driving south from Chania airport, I watch her soak it up.

And the village has a special welcome. A resident and mischievous pelican, fresh from its favourite pastime of dive-bombing people swimming in the shallows, comes waddling purposefully towards us.

Emma is astonished, fearful almost, and can hardly believe it is real. She has only seen pelicans in a book before, and when it takes off, its wing-span almost filling the narrow cobbled street, she turns to look at me in amazement.

That evening, although she is withdrawn and the night is spent almost in silence, she is reflective at this point, rather than troubled:

*Many happy and wondrous moments today. Wishing I didn't have language, so I could just 'drink' in the views around me, pure sight, no complication of thought . . . Glad to be on holiday at last.*

The following day, however, Emma's demons emerge to plague her. Away from the stress and the familiarity of London and of moving into the flat, there is time here for her to be faced with the troubles she carries inside her which have not been left behind:

*Yesterday i found myself in the view of the rocks, the wave-crested sea, the mountains . . . i found myself in the enormous starry sky seen from the beach. Today i found myself in some small beautiful stones along the beach . . . i did not find myself in other people.*

The alienation I feel in Emma, which locks me out, casts me aside, and which takes the form of sullenness, arrogance even, is here with us in Crete, in this beautiful place I had hoped might melt her wish to cut herself off from life.

On a walk up into the hills to Anidri, to spend time in a tiny church with Byzantine murals covering part of the walls, she is especially difficult. I ask for directions and, a few hundred yards further on, am not sure of the way again.

Pausing to look back, to try and work it out, Emma is impatient with me and demands:

'What are we waiting for?'

'I'm not sure where the left turn is they told us to take.'

'Weren't you listening to what they said?' she scolds, as if I were a wayward child.

'Weren't you? There are two of us here.'

But Emma is not really with me. Our lovely surroundings have had a deeply unsettling effect on her. Startlingly beautiful as they are, they strip her of something. They do not provide her with a reason to be angry and they unlock a dread in her that it is only she, Emma, who is bad and wrong.

On the way back down the hill, stopping for a moment on a bend in the road, I say how beautiful it is and she falls apart.

'I can't bear it,' she sobs, 'when all this is so beautiful and I feel so bad.'

That evening is pleasant, though. We sit in a harbour restaurant having an early drink and, reminding me of the pebbles on the beach in Brighton, Emma wants to know how long she is allowed to sit by the sea looking at stones, to lose herself in this way. She is happy doing this, she says, and knows she could do it for a long time. But she is by herself and is this OK, to have this kind of solitary happiness?

I sigh. One of the aspects of being with Emma I find difficult is the sound of my own voice in long explanations. It troubles me. Stories are fine, but expositions feel wearying, preachy, and not what life is about.

She needs to learn to have some, not all, of something, I suggest. We all do. Many people fear their appetites, for pleasure, for work, as well as for food. So it isn't just her. It is a question of balance.

I suggest, then, that she should spend more spontaneous time with people, just saying hello and a few words, especially local people here, who are friendly. She could buy our fruit and groceries, talk to people in the shops.

It is the 'people thing' which frightens her, she says, looking doubtful.

Yes. Stones stay still and do not answer back. That is why people are more of a challenge.

She tells me that when she catches sight of her reflection in a shop window it is like a knife in her heart.

Why?

Because it's not a nice picture. She looks horrible.

She closes herself off, I say, makes herself look sullen:

'You don't have to do this. You know how to be loving – you were, with me, as a child. But you stopped.'

Emma's accolades are rare at any time so I am surprised when she says, suddenly, how amazing it is that she knows me, just because she said 'hello' to me in a pub.

Imagine what her life would be like if she had not done this.

But the rest of the holiday is difficult, relieved only, for me, by unexpectedly meeting a colleague from years back, sitting with his girlfriend in a restaurant. He, she and I spend a day or two together. Emma is invited of course but does not come. She is busy eating.

I catch her doing it when, out for the evening, it suddenly turns chilly and I go back for a sweater. Opening the door, Emma is high on refined sugar, like someone on drugs, babbling, confessing. She deliberately missed supper, then bought bars of chocolate, binged them all and threw up.

I am in despair, my fervent, and perhaps foolish, hope that this holiday, this beautiful place, would soothe and help Emma, dashed. At a loss what to do, it is Emma who comes up with a practical solution.

Although mainly we eat out, our flat is self-catering with breakfast stuff, fruit and bread kept in a cupboard – all of which is now removed and, at Emma's request, kept under my bed where she believes she will not rummage for it. My turn to feel surreal.

The following day is easier, spent watching the pelican at play. Shrieks from round the harbour as it dive-bombs swimmers. Emma swims far out, staying in the water a long time. I am afraid after a while, swimming out to look for her. What if she does not come back?

The following morning, the fifth day into our week, produces a bright, starry start to a trip to the Samaria Gorge. I am excited, having wanted to walk the gorge for some time.

Near the top, before the difficult descent over large stones worn slippery like glass by hundreds of thousands of footsteps, Emma asks, suddenly: 'Am I hungry? Should I have something to eat?'

And I realise she, her body, is so confused, she probably has no way of knowing whether she needs food or not, whether she wants to eat because her mouth or her obsession wants to, or because she is genuinely hungry.

Set meal-times which the Unit has asked her to follow stop this, of course, but Emma has blown this regime a long while before we came on holiday.

As she blows the rest of the walk without me. Euphoric, perhaps binge-eating, I am not sure, she sails through the long walk on her own, in soft-soled shoes through which the stones must surely hurt her feet.

Returning to Gatwick, standing waiting for the Victoria train, Emma asks insistent questions: what time will the train arrive; which platform does it go from; how many stops does it take?
We travel in silence.

# Chapter Thirty-One

## A Lot of Noise

It has not occurred to me that, to get her housed, Emma is classified as mentally ill and has been given accommodation set aside for people with mental health problems. It has not occurred to her either. And she is furious when the young men upstairs, one of whom has schizophrenia, start making a noise and shouting late at night, eventually banging on her door.

I hope she didn't open it, I venture anxiously.

Oh, yes she did, she says. She was ready for them by this time, absolutely furious. She needs her sleep and gave them a large wedge of her mind:

'You two are annoying me,' she had shouted at them. 'Now go away and don't bother me again.'

They take to leaving black rubbish bags outside her back door for her to trip over as she comes out, as do the people who live in the house next door. Not prepared to have

'weirdos' living next to them, when Emma, at my suggestion, goes to talk to them, the man who answers the door
shouts:

'You're all mad in that house. Now clear off.'

Emma handles this surprisingly well. But the problems
she has with her mother are never far away. Although she
has not seen Colleen for months, her clothes and belongings are still 'at home' and Emma has keys to the house.

Feeling unsettled by her holiday in Crete, by her own
behaviour, and by how difficult she found being away, she
uses her keys the day after we return, to go in, raid the
cupboards for food, binge-eat and be sick.

In her diary she writes of the familiarity of 'the glistening green bowl' and the note on the bathroom water heater:
'Ensure that the system is thoroughly flushed out.'

Colleen comes in as Emma is leaving the bathroom and
says nothing.

'She acted as if nothing had happened,' Emma says. 'There
were food packets all over the place. She must have known.'

Emma's therapist and dietician are both away at this
time and, what with black binbags on her doorstep, trying
to settle into living on her own, and me being busy with
work, she has little support. Nevertheless, I take issue with
her. What she, Emma, did at her parents' home was aggressive, to herself as well as to her mother. And, realistically,
what does she expect Colleen to do? What does she want?
She knows her mother will not, cannot, accept the extent
of Emma's pain and distress. And Emma has left home.

'I feel angry with her for existing,' Emma says at one point and then, at another, feeling contrite, that she thought she had left Colleen behind when she left her parents' house and how this is not so. The problems are still with her, she realises, deep inside, and what is she to do?

Emma is exhausting at this time, throwing a panoply of emotional states at me which I find almost impossible to deal with.

I remember something I had meant to ask her following a conversation with a friend who is a mental health adviser. Talking to him about Emma's continuing poor state, I tell him about our trip to Crete, and the morning on the steps of the Samaria Gorge, when Emma had not known whether she was hungry or not.

What does Jim think of this? Is it Emma fooling me or is it genuine, her not knowing the difference, after so much abuse, between real hunger and the need to eat constantly? Jim asks me to get Emma to check what anti-depressants she is on. He is certain the people at the Unit will have thought of it, but there is no harm in double-checking: some anti-depressants suppress the part of the brain which tells you whether or not you are hungry.

So, with her therapist returning the following week, I mention this to Emma, who is furious – and anxious.

No, she is not going to check it, she says, her anti-depressants are not that sort.

How does she know?

Because she eats whether she is hungry or not. She always knows when she is *really* hungry.

But there was the time in Crete when she asked me about it, about whether or not she needed food.

No she did not. She never said that. Wouldn't say it. Didn't ask. She is shouting by now.

Bluntly I say I do not tell her things that are not true, and she crumples.

She is sorry, she says tearfully and, going over to where she is sitting on the settee, holding her as she weeps, she then tells me what is *really* wrong:

'I can't see my mother. I daren't see her, and it hurts so much. I don't think I can bear it.'

I barely think I can either, Emma looking so fragile and unable to manage, and I wonder how this can possibly be resolved – Emma's tremendous need for Colleen to witness her pain and to join in her repair.

Emma still wants to be able to hurt Colleen, to lash out, be sick in her bathroom, enough to know she matters, and that, whatever she does, Colleen will still accept her.

While Colleen does stay constant to Emma, never refusing her a home, she keeps herself at a distance, which leaves Emma feeling stranded. Having declared herself an orphan, Emma is not happy enough, strong enough, capable enough, to survive on her own.

Colleen is still the central place of Emma's longed-for comfort, and of her unplaced love, and listening to Emma, talking to her, holding her when she cries, I see how this flat is only the beginning of her wish for a home of her own. Now she is facing the mother *inside*.

Eventually, as she quietens, I say her pain will not go on for ever. She is brave to face it and it will ease and what about Paul? Does she talk to him?

Wiping tears from her face, she nods.

Well that is a good thing, then. And isn't it marvellous that he can love both her mother and her. That is really something to build on, and to be glad about. She should speak to him as often as she needs to.

But the next six weeks are awful. Emma is distressed and angry and then there are her sighs on the phone and her silences, her need for me to talk and talk, and find the right words for her time and time again when I am already exhausted by this.

She is like a sponge, soaking up my carefully chosen sentences, just listening as I plead, cajole, insist, inform. I tell her there was a reason for her illness, that neither her mother, nor her father, were able to give her what she genuinely needed. These things happen. She is not a bad person, doomed to have a bad life. And so it goes on, until the next time.

Things start to improve a little, beginning with her telling me about her feet one day. She has injured them, she says. I am flummoxed. What does she mean, injured her feet? How?

Stamping on the floor she tells me. It is what she does to vent her anger. She stamps.

Well, I am glad she has the downstairs flat in that case, I say wryly. I would not like her feet thumping over *my* head.

She laughs and asks if I would like to see Stomp with her at the Roundhouse in Camden Town.

Looking better when I see her a few days later at my place, she is getting her anger out, she tells me. She found Dawn from Community Care had been in her flat again, moving things around, and she was so angry . . .

Ooh, not her feet . . .

Shaking her head. No, not her feet. She went into the bedroom and smacked pillows at the wall for five minutes. That did the trick. Keen to demonstrate, she takes me out into the hallway, where she flings a pillow from my bed against the wall opposite. It makes a noise like a rifle shot.

I am astonished. So, what did she do with her feet, then, to hurt them? Just show me once. No more. And I flinch as she shoves her foot into the floor, like a fist piling into an enemy's face. What must it do to her spine?

I far prefer the pillow trick, I say, and, putting it back on the bed, we are ready to go out for the night.

'Carpet-beating must have been so satisfying,' she says wistfully as we walk down the stairs.

She enjoys the show, a heady mix of noise; energy; percussion; dance; improvisation. Driving her to the nearest tube afterwards, she is alive, enthusiastic and says how much she would like to do work like that herself.

'It would *really* give them something to complain about upstairs,' she says with a giggle.

She looks young, happy and, watching her leave, her long coat trailing, floppy hat flapping in the breeze, she seems like any other twenty-year-old. Turning to wave to me, she looks vulnerable, too, trusting, and I want to shout something about being sure to take care of herself. I want to tell her that she matters to me.

But I let her go.

# Chapter Thirty-Two

᚜

## VOICES FROM AFAR

Emma's longings and distress over her dealings with her mother continue. Now that she is in a flat of her own, Colleen has been phoning her to see how she is getting along, and Emma has had Paul and her mother over to show them her new place and cook them a meal.

She spent ages preparing, she tells me, and it went really, really well, but she says no more and I think it best not to ask. For there is something about what she has said, or the way she says it, which does not ring true.

Emma's feelings of hurt and disappointment when she sees Colleen persist. She needs such a lot from her mother and, unwittingly, when Colleen is nonchalant, perhaps, or busy, or simply being herself, Emma feels set back. She continues to yearn for the fantasy mother she wants Colleen to be.

At one point Emma writes she wants to mean 'everything

to <u>someone</u>'. This is after a phonecall from Colleen, which distressed Emma because her mother was 'ordinary' and Emma, feeling desperately needy, wanted so much more:

> I nearly had a panic attack when my mother rang . . . wanting to knead my body like a lump of raw dough, knead it, roll it, the big pale fat mound of meat, shapeless and tasteless and repulsive. Slice into the flesh, beat it . . . kill it . . .
>
> I want to burrow down into my own private little hole in the ground, and hibernate for all eternity . . . Life's dangerous and painful and scary.

Unbeknown to me, but recorded in her diaries, Emma is continuing to binge and vomit, her weight rising from nine stone before we went to Crete in September, to around ten stone or more in the couple of months since then.

Going to the Unit as a day-patient presents difficulties too. She forms intense friendships with other girls and is hurt and fiercely jealous if she thinks someone else is more friendly with a girl she wants to be friends with, or if she is left out of conversations.

She and I see each other as usual. I go to her flat, have her round to mine, take her out. Stand by. But living on her own, facing the routine of a daily life, is proving almost too much for her when this seemingly ordinary arrangement is so at odds with the maelstrom of emotion inside her: rage; longing; hope; despair and, I have recently discovered, depression.

When we came back from Crete and I questioned her about them, it was news to me that Emma was on antidepressants. She has never mentioned them.

When I ask her, now, she says simply that she has been on and off them for a few years, since going to the Unit. Since it is clear this is all she wants to say, I leave it there.

To try and give her life some structure, there are practical suggestions I make, that she returns to a dance class or joins a music class, to meet other people and enjoy herself. And the Alexander Technique might help with her relationship with her body. I find her someone, Claire, who is just qualified, whom Emma sees for quite a while.

She works a few hours in a local charity shop, and I think that might be good too. She likes helping people, and it may strengthen her.

So, she does what she can, and in between the despair which her diary speaks of at this time, there are flashes of hope, like the days when her eating is 'gloriously normal'. And there are other hopes too:

*I want to meet a wonderful man and fall in love. I want what everyone else wants, so I guess I'm not really so strange after all. Life can be wonderful sometimes, and sometimes it almost even makes sense.*

She also records the beginning of her wish to do something with her life and be someone in the world:

*Social life growing. <u>Craving</u> for academic life. <u>I want something to be passionate about</u>. I want to do something . . . wanting to go to museums and galleries and to learn. Wanting to read intelligent, powerful, important, life-changing books.*

When she comes to my place, Emma scours my bookshelves for poetry, drama, fiction, polemic. We go to films together and I tell her stories, still. She asks me to repeat the ones about her stays in my place: her tidying the house; the whistling wigeon; and do I still hear from King Alfred?

At home, in her flat, local people from Community Care still come in when she is not around to check on the place. She has asked for this to stop, or for it to happen while she is there, but people are busy, and the rules are clear. While she is in this kind of accommodation, Dawn or someone like her, has the key:

*Yesterday, someone was in my flat. I arrived home and was absolutely <u>livid</u> and used the ultimate expression of my anger – slapping the pillow hard with all my force against the wall to create an almighty THWACK.*

*One of the upstairs neighbours came down and was*

*banging at the front door, but I ignored him. It's not often I make noise, and five minutes of noisy wallslapping is a much healthier solution than four hours of bingeing and vomiting . . .*

*In time I know I'll need to find a quieter way to vent my anger, but for now I'm enjoying this way too much to change.*

Emma seems to be finding a vantage point for her illness at last, somewhere to see it from, some perspective:

*Anorexia is so cruel, devastating, evil, mindless, volatile, unforgiving, relentless, despairing, powerful, dominating, suffocating, choking, murderous, to blame, horrific, hateful, degrading, manipulative . . .*

*Anorexia has no word to describe its full horror. The full horror is visual – embodied in the anorexic, creeping, creeping, ever onwards, into the only future she can see – where in the world of floating ghosts, it's she who reigns supreme.*

*I'm going to fight against anorexia with all my might – I want to kick up an <u>enormous</u> fuss, alert people . . . Women are dying, slowly killing themselves as the world sits back complacently and watches them parade their adorned corpses down catwalks, glazed eyes and false smiles . . . it's so wrong, and I want to change it . . . I need to find my voice, and a way to get it heard.*

Emma still looks well and happy when, at her request, we meet on Christmas Eve at my place to go to St Paul's Cathedral for a family carol service beginning at four o'clock. It is one I go to most years and, hearing me talk of it, Emma has asked to come too.

I am amazed she has never been to St Paul's, not even seen the outside of the building nor sat in the peace of the gardens.

She looks lovely. Her skin is clear of the face-picking she still sometimes indulges in and she is happy to be with me. Both with our hats and long coats, it is only Emma who has thought to bring an umbrella, which we share as it begins to rain. Arm in arm, we walk the mile or so from the Angel down through back streets, old alleyways and courtyards, to the vast wooden doors of St Paul's.

She thinks it is wonderful, squeezes my arm, shakes her head gently, almost in disbelief. All these people, thousands of them, and she looks, feels, safe and warm.

As the congregation settles into quietness for the service to begin, from a distant arm of the cathedral, invisible to us for now, one lone choirboy sings the first note of the first carol.

Far off to begin with, the choir begins to move along this outer wing of the building, its voices imperceptibly becoming fuller as the choristers walk slowly towards the main body of the cathedral.

Into view at last, the carol nearing its end, I feel, as perhaps we all do, that the song, and we, have already travelled a long, peaceful way.

It is a beautiful service. St Paul's is welcoming as always and, going in at dusk, it is night by the time we emerge onto the steps to the pealing of bells round London, and it is truly Christmas Eve.

Curled up in armchairs at my place a little later, before Emma goes back to her flat, and then to her parents' for Christmas Day, we talk about the year almost gone, and about how far she has come back towards life from the lonely place of her illness.

It has been harder than she would ever have imagined, this long journey, but she has, among other things, moved into a place of her own and discovered the frustration, as well as the freedom, that has involved. She has taken up singing lessons, and has begun the courageous task of facing her anger.

She has, too, a growing ability to join in and to share with others, to accept being part of life. Her voice, small and far away to begin with, is becoming stronger, fuller, closer to being heard.

# Chapter Thirty-Three

## COMING OUT

Living on her own, finding it difficult to draw on inner resources, Emma decides she needs to be stronger and writes in her diaries of wanting stronger friends.

In beginning to turn her back on anorexia, sadly she knows she will have to stop relying on the friends she has made at the Unit, where she continues to go as a day-patient. She is further along the road of repair and retrieval than they are and they hold her back:

> *They cannot be the friends I need as long as they are unwell . . . I need to be around stronger people, and it hurts so much to know this . . . things are changed within, and suddenly everything is different, you can't go back.*

So Emma goes forward: into being more involved in the

world outside the Unit; into going to art galleries; catching buses and tubes; walking in parks; taking care of herself; learning to live a life. She meets different people and, out clubbing, she begins to enjoy dancing again and men's company:

> *so this is life. It's nice, in a beautifully twisted sort of way. And this is what I've been hiding from all my life. It's not so bad after all, being normal, being alive . . . It gave me a lot of pleasure when Oliver told me that I have a great body . . .*

Alongside these up-beat times, Emma feels lost and invisible in the crowds moving along London's streets. The depression which dogs her makes it almost impossible, on some days, for her to do anything.

Like the night I go over in January 1999. She has promised to cook me supper and, when I arrive, there is nothing prepared. She is listless, despondent and I am hungry.

I can understand her spells of extreme lowness, for she is twenty years old and has missed more than five years of her life to the acute form of her illness and even more if you count the way it was affecting her, in the background, long before.

Anorexia has kept her down, under and away from life. Under the guise of keeping her safe from scary and uncontrollable events, it has removed her from competence and the experience gained from daily living. It has retarded her.

The aspect of life Emma finds frightening and writes of so often is that you have to take risks.

Being unpossessed of the ability easily to do so, her fall-back position has been illness. Rather than be adventurous, she has retired to a place somewhere between health and disease, between life and death: the trance-like state of her subliminal preoccupation with food.

In February, visiting Emma again, she has gained at least half a stone in the three weeks since last I saw her. The weight is too new, has been put on too fast and is worrying, therefore. It looks uneven and her face is spotty from where she has been picking at it.

But her flat looks lovely. Vases of tulips, and white roses in a long triangular vase, a bookcase in her bedroom and pictures on the walls: one of her as a three-year-old in a red top looking inquisitive, determined – and sweet.

There is the one of her and me at my fortieth, she in red again, head down studying a chocolate box I am holding for her. There is a recent one of her and her mother, Emma looking mightily pleased to have her arm round Colleen, the latter reserving judgement, though, giving nothing away either to Emma or the camera.

Her flat is well cared for, lived in and tidy, except in the bedroom where what I call the 'tyrannical' toys of her childhood are massed: a furry army, dozens of soft toys crammed into the bookshelf and round the wardrobe.

They have always disturbed me. Substitutes for love is how I view them, Emma's bedroom crammed with them since childhood, the things she was bought which were supposed to make her happy. But they have been her company for a long time, and I say nothing about them.

Asking how she has been she says not good. She cannot find a shape to her life and is worried about what career she might take up. She has an appointment with a careers adviser in a week or so to discuss it. She is interested in child psychology but is that a good thing for her to do? How will she make up her mind?

Next month, she is leaving the Unit as a day-patient, she tells me, and is leaving her therapist, too.

Not wanting to sound alarmist, I ask if there will be back-up. Will she be able to phone her therapist if she needs to?

No, she says, it is a clean break.

I am concerned for her. She has only been getting better for a few months. And without so many ordinary experiences, those of having lived what would be called a 'normal' life, where she would have learned to grow and develop and, especially, to take risks and make mistakes, she is unprepared, I fear, to be left on her own.

Not hearing from her, after a few days I ring to see how she is.

'Weird' is her answer. 'Feeling a bit weird.'

She is missing the Unit, not as it is now, because it's changed a lot in the last year – as has she in relation to it – but as it was a year ago.

This concerns me, for a year ago she was badly ill.

Is there any contact with the Unit? Does she go and visit?

Yes, she sees a doctor once a month and yes, in answer to my question, the doctor is someone she could ask for more therapy and back-up if she needed it.

But is she still seeing people, doing things?

Her diary reveals:

> *I'm drained, exhausted . . . postponing things, refusing to think about things . . . a prison of stillness.*

It is almost genetically imprinted, a parent's need, as well as wish, for a child to be happy, not just for the child's sake, but for the adult who does the caring. There is a need for an unhappy or sick child whose bedside you have sat by to pull through. You want something, someone, at the end of the hours, weeks – years – of 'holding on'.

After years of helping, I do not want Emma to give up – for my sake as well as hers. I want Emma to 'make it', for her to be competent and well. For there is something going on in her at this time which makes me fearful: she is at a crisis point in the distressing level of her feelings about Colleen.

Emma is almost beside herself, the size of her emotions frightening her, the fact that she wants her mother desperately and at the same time is furious with her. And, as her substitute mother, she is furious, by proxy, with me.

Visiting her in her flat, aggression is on the rampage like poison gas seeping out of the sofa she is sitting on. She glares at me. Even when we are discussing the people upstairs, or the rubbish bags, her gaze is huge, furious, devouring, and I have nowhere to put my eyes. I can only look down or away.

However, amazingly, tenaciously, she is looking for college A-level courses to begin getting the qualifications she needs to go to university. I encourage her and I think, as before, not just about the pieces of paper she might gain, but the new friends.

Having met a few of Emma's friends – a couple when she was a young teenager and a few on the Unit who, like her, have been ill – I have wanted her to meet new people, have the chance to find the stronger friends her diaries speak of.

I implore her to phone me, to let me help her choose a course, but she does not ring, nor come round. She is back to the dangerous place of wanting, needing, demanding, I go to her.

There are many 'misses' between Emma and Colleen at this time: talks on the phone; miscommunication; thwarted hopes.

Visiting her in March, her mother was here, Emma tells me, the two of them by themselves. Emma told Colleen she had recovered from her anorexia now, and was leaving the Unit and setting out to live a normal life.

Emma tells me her mother said she did not know if it

was true that Emma was recovered. She was not sure about this. Was Emma mistaken or lying still?

Her recovery fragile, Emma plummeted after this: binge-eating; staying in bed; getting up late; picking her face again.

I cannot know what happened between them, whether it was Emma being defensive, giving her impression of being self-contained.

Or was Emma saying, gladly, like a child showing off to a mother, that she was on the way to being well again?

For Colleen's part, was she simply concerned about Emma, seeing through the façade she presented, and trying to bring her down to earth? Or was *she* being defensive?

But, as she tells me about Colleen's visit, Emma is sobbing, clinging to me as she cries:

'I can't see my mother. Not for a long time. It hurts too much. It's too dangerous.'

And neither, for a while, does she see me.

Without either of us knowing it, Emma has reached a place which she would most want to avoid. Her need for the safety of the illness she knows so well is matched by the reality that she has engaged too much with the world, responded to it, 'tasted' it too often, to go back. Life has grabbed her and in the battle between 'Big Life', as she calls it, and anorexia, the former is winning. For the tug, the force of life is too strong for Emma to resist.

Yet, she tries to resist, for living is still painful and difficult for her and bulimia beckons, dragging her the other way.

Professional help withdrawn to a minimum, she gets worse it seems. Ten bars of chocolate, binge-eating every day, depression, self-hatred.

Whenever I see her, she looks as if she wants to over-power or devour me with her eyes, which are filled with fury, and I cannot, should not, have to bear this.

Not knowing how far out of her illness she has come, I believe, instead, she may be on the point of regressing. I cannot deal with it and 'crash' myself.

I cannot go through another of Emma's loops. It would be too much for me. If she is heading towards anorexia again, I have nothing left to give.

It has been almost five years since I first heard she was seriously ill in a hospital bed and went racing to her that sunny afternoon.

In those years, I have worried about her, cared for her, tried to deal, practically, with the grave proportions of her unpossession and I have been angry with anorexia on her behalf.

Now I am angry with *her*. If she is going to treat me badly, I will not accept it. A reference she wants me to write for an A-level course is, ironically, the straw which breaks me.

Why don't you come over? I ask, when she rings about it. We can do it together.

'Oh, I'm too busy for that,' she says airily.

Doing what?

Oh, seeing friends, shopping, this and that.

Well, in that case, I am busy too. Telling her perfunctorily that I will have it ready for her to pick up in a few days' time, she demurs: couldn't I put it in the post?

No. She can pick it up.

When she does, I hand her the unsealed reference to read. It says that while Emma is more than bright enough to take the course, she is just recovering from a long period of anorexia and would need help, in the form of counselling or support of some kind, to sustain her.

She is furious. How dare I say something like that.

Because, in my opinion, it is true. Now, if she will excuse me, I have things to do . . .

# Chapter Thirty-Four

~§

## THE LETTER TO HER MIRROR

For two months, there is silence. I am sad, first of all, regretful, and then relieved. Emma's illness has been a burden on me for far too long.

Friends had warned I should have protected myself more against what one wise person called the 'involuntary greed' of people who are ill in the way Emma has been.

Her demands on me *have* felt like greed at times. At others, they have drawn on my affection for her – 'pulled at my heart-strings' – in a way which has made it difficult for me not to respond.

Have I responded too much I wonder. Have I given too much? The hard work of educating Emma out of her unpossessed state has been time-consuming and difficult, involving high quality 'feeding on demand'. All those answers to Emma's questions: what knife and fork to use; which hand to hold the fork in if you're eating with a fork only; what to say if someone is rude to you; what to say to a boy you like; how to wash and care for yourself.

So how does she change, she wants to know in the months leading up to me deciding I have had enough. What does it involve?

And how can we move on from all this? I wonder. It is such a strange thing to have done, to have sat for hours, over weeks and months, helping her catch up. Cramming for life.

Emma gone for now, the phone silent, I look again at *Internal Landscapes*, Gianna Williams's book on anorexia. She writes that people suffering from the illness have 'highly impervious defences to ward off the experience of need and dependency'. It makes sense. If you deny the need for food, you do not have to feel dependent on anyone for you have not taken anything from them.

So, the part of Emma which wants to be my equal, or even my superior, which says airily that she is busy, and wishes to deny me my place in her life, seems to me to be the aspect of her which does not want to accept I have done anything for her – or to rely on me.

She does not want to admit she is dependent. Instead, she accepts what I have to offer as if it means nothing. And the more, of late, I have given, filling her up with 'food for life', the more she has wanted, both to take what I have had to give and to deny any 'debt' she might feel she owes me.

It is not indebtedness I want from Emma, though, but recognition for being who I am, and for caring about her.

In May, the message on my answerphone says she has missed me and would like to meet. Her voice has changed. No longer strained, or pretending to be indifferent, she sounds balanced and well.

At my place a few days later she is happy and affectionate. It is a sunny day and, in reminiscing mode, we walk by the canal. Emma tells me friends of hers, and a new friend – a boyfriend? – called Simon, have been telling her how horribly she has been behaving. She has been really awful to be with, they have told her, and she realises she was foul to me and she is sorry.

Relieved to hear I was not the only person Emma was foul to, I enjoy listening to her again as she talks of her time with me as a child and how much it meant to her: feeding the ducks; cooking make-believe cakes in the hut in the park; not minding getting wet if it rained; splashing in puddles; laughing a lot; sitting in together, warm and happy.

'Am I still your favourite girl?' she asks, with a smile.

I feel easier about Emma in the months which follow. Yes, Simon is a boyfriend, and they come for tea. I like him and it is a pleasure to see them together holding hands, chatting openly, smiling at each other.

They get themselves fed a lot – home cooking. Every Friday they go to his parents, and every Saturday or Sunday to Emma's. So they see Colleen and Paul every week, and Emma enjoys her parents more. She feels relaxed with them at last, now that she has Simon on her side.

In between, Emma and Simon come to my place for

food – and I visit theirs. There is something disturbing, though, about Simon's flat. Emma has colonised it and I cannot see a masculine object or corner in the whole place. The walls, shelves, surfaces are full of Emma's girly objects – furry animals, trinkets, hearts, cards, flowery things. It is overwhelmingly sugary.

I should stop worrying, I tell myself. But, as it turns out, Simon suffers badly from depression and by the end of the year he is in hospital, and they have split up.

Telling me about it on the phone, Emma is low again. It was she who ended it, she says. Simon was getting jealous and possessive, and had started shouting at her. Soon after, it became clear that he was clinically depressed.

She had visited him in hospital, but she could not get through to him and it became too upsetting. But now that she is on her own, she still misses him terribly, and feels confused and lonely. To get herself through this difficult period, Emma decides to return to therapy, which Colleen pays for.

By Christmas of that year, Emma has said goodbye to her illness. In her diary, in a long, formal and dramatic letter entitled 'Dear anorexia and bulimia', she writes, as if to a lover, of the years she has been involved with them both:

*I once held you close . . . Anorexia . . . Your cold white dwelling was my home, my retreat, my release, and I adored its empty halls, its cool blank* walls. Perfectly smooth, immaculate, untouched, clean, serene, quiet, silent, desolate, alone. The world I used to live in, exist in, try to survive in, nearly died in . . .

Holding your cold hand, feeling your icy breath skate along my spine . . .

Wild rampant hunger driving me on and up and away into a higher state, the rush of emptying out a gorged stomach . . . until fatigue ended the feast . . .

I can now be touched by joy, by pain . . .; I can make mistakes, and accept change. I can laugh until my stomach aches . . . give . . . take, and I can break apart. I can feel . . . I can see all the colours of the rainbow . . . and I can live without you, at last.

She concludes:

I needed you to get through each fragile day. You were my adventure, my melodrama . . . my lover, my destiny, my fate . . . Part of me now has died with you, and I want to cry for the girl I was then . . . and I never want to forget she was me. I'm scared that I'll forget her. Her and me.

# Chapter Thirty-Five

❦

## Remembering

In early 2000, Emma is in her second term of an A-level course, this time in Psychology. As with her first attempt at A-levels, she is taking two years to do this one subject. It is what she can manage as she learns to 'come out', to be with other people and adjust to life, all at the same time.

Not taking on too much is also a way of defending herself against a problem with her memory. It used to be very good and now it is patchy at times. This can make her seem inattentive and remote as she struggles to fill in the gaps. Talking to her about it, she says:

'I remember how it was before I was ill and there's a definite difference. Studying was easier before. I could retain facts and vocabulary easily. Concepts are still fine. I can grasp them, but it bothers me a lot that it's harder to study and to remember other things too.

'I don't remember to tell people things – about what I've done. I'll be talking to a friend about going out, say, and forget to say something really important that happened which I wanted to say all along.'

Since medical experts I speak to say there is usually no permanent memory loss as a result of the anorexia, I suggest Emma talks to a doctor about it. For she is coping with a lot at this time. As well as difficulty with studying, Emma is in mourning for the predictable habits of the illness which have engulfed her for so many years. They are what she has known and she feels lost, naked, without them – lonely.

She does what she can to catch up, to learn how to be in 'Big Life', rather than the cut-off world of anorexia, but her first year or two 'out' are immensely hard. Not only the catching up, but her sense of self. For, without the identity of her illness, who is she?

*Most of the time I just feel helpless, small, and stupid.*

Then, an urge to speed things up:

*I want to try a new dance class. I want to do kick-boxing . . . boxercise . . . I want to learn about the world – sociology, economics, theology, philosophy, cultural studies, psychology . . . historical studies – so much brain food. I'm eager, so eager to drink in as much knowledge as I possibly can.*

But how to match this with Emma's slowness and her struggle to study? In order to reduce life to a pace where she can manage it, she has been slow for many years, she tells me. She has had so little energy, almost since she can remember, and everything has, therefore, been an effort for her.

In her renewed efforts to engage more directly with her surroundings, Emma tries to be less defensive with people:

*I am trying hard to be more open with friends about myself and my insecurities . . .*

She also notices her meanness with herself. She has, after all, lived a cut-down version of life, where she has not had to think about ordinary things like buying clothes, for example:

*I find it difficult to spend money on myself . . . I don't pay to have my hair trimmed any more, I haven't had a proper pair of shoes since I don't know when — I want to start appreciating myself a bit more . . . I'm very tired.*

Doing what she can to address her needs, but also needing time to grieve for the illness she seems to have left behind, Emma returns for a while to dressing plainly, frumpily even, and takes little pride in her appearance.

An important part of Emma's determination to return to life at this time is her improved relationship with her mother. This repair is obvious from comments here and there. When I ask after Colleen and Paul she will tell me they are fine. They still watch football and go for walks with the dog.

Does she talk to Colleen more now?

'Well, yes and no.' Then, with a wry smile: 'You know how Mum is. Communication's not her strong point.'

Although it has been difficult for Emma to know what to expect from her mother, she has changed from wanting everything from Colleen to being able to accept, more, who her mother is. And she needs Colleen less.

Through going to college, making new friends, and finding, after their break-up, a new relationship, a strong friendship, with Simon, she finds, at last, a feeling of 'normality' and independence and no longer has the need to hurt Colleen.

Talking about it, one day while we are shopping for clothes and having a coffee in between, Emma says: 'I always wanted something from her and I used to think she didn't give it to me deliberately. So I was hurt.

'Now I understand she didn't give it to me because that isn't how she is.'

Relieved of the pressure of wanting something, everything, from Colleen, she thinks about what life might have been like for her mother:

'At the time I felt she didn't want me around, didn't care. She was at work all day and when she came home she wanted time on her own, to relax and didn't want a kid hanging round her asking questions, wanting to play and things like that.'

Emma says she believes, now, that Colleen was not ready for this:

'I don't think she was ready to be a mother because she wasn't ready to make sacrifices. There were some she *did* make, but she wasn't ready to sacrifice time to spend with me. And she wasn't ready, or maybe she didn't know how, to show affection, show me that she loved me.'

In having a better relationship with Colleen, Emma comes to enjoy me again, too. We have meals together quite often and her mouth has changed. No longer eating inwardly, it is not twisted any more, in thrall to the thought of bingeing or starvation.

There are other things, too. Emma enjoys her food at last and, believing her tastebuds to have been execrably treated by years of neglect and excess, I enjoy cooking tasty meals for her and spending time at the table chatting as we eat. Emma tells me later how important this was to her:

'You helped me see eating as something obviously normal and OK to get pleasure from. You were the only person who showed me that.'

As she continues to grow stronger, Emma asks to borrow my green dress, the one I took to Vienna, for a wedding reception she and Simon are going to. Although she and

I are different sizes, it fits. We are different colourings too – me dark, her fair – but the frock can take us both.

This dress hanging in my wardrobe has been a beckoning object between Emma and me – a piece of silk with a story attached, retrieved from the time of her despair and wafting through into the present. For when she was still ill, Emma and I would look at my clothes together, symbols as they were of a life lived out in the world. There were 'stories' attached to many of these garments which she had enjoyed listening to.

'Could I wear something like this?' she would ask, about a linen skirt or a hand-painted blouse.

Yes.

Taking the green frock out of its dustproof wrapping, she had said: 'Ooh, isn't this gorgeous. The material. It's lovely. Could I borrow this if I got better?'

Yes, of course.

Emma continues to grow in the world, to accept how it is and what is has to offer her. Having swapped the predictable mirror of anorexia for the 'no guarantees', 'in your face' nature of real life, she grimaces now and then and is not deterred. As the months go by, she starts taking more of an interest in buying clothes for herself. We shop, sometimes. She laughs more.

In the spring of 2001, a few months before Emma sits her psychology exam, I have a party to launch my latest book. Dozens of people come to celebrate in the upstairs room of an old London pub, Emma and Simon among them.

I feel ridiculously proud of them both: Simon, who likes being casual, dressed up specially in a suit; and Emma looking lovely in a long frock, both of them smiling – and with a bouquet of flowers for me.

Friends who know Emma say how well she looks, how marvellously happy, and people who have never met them say how lovely they both are.

They mingle easily, are surrounded by people, I notice, as I watch out for them during the early part of the evening. They obviously enjoy themselves.

Two musician friends, Chris on double bass and Pete on guitar, have offered to play and sing for a few hours and, towards the end of the evening I see Emma is on the dais with them. As the room hushes she says in her soft, but clear, voice that she would like to sing me a song.

Seemingly undaunted by the large gathering, she tells us that when she stayed in my house as a little girl, we played this record a lot and danced together. It is one of our favourites, she says, with a smile in my direction.

Emma's voice. I will always enjoy it: its fullness, soft-ness, clarity, and the gentleness I hear so often, now, on the phone. I have heard it through all its ranges: cracked; husky; furious; despairing in these awful years she has been through; and, at times, nearly taken from me, nearly gone. Tears running down my face, I listen to the girl who was afraid to sing, fill the room.

A long number, it surprises me now, as it did when she was a child, how much she liked Don McLean's 'American

Pie', and asked for it to be played every time she came round. Is that why she has remembered so much of it?

The room silent for her, the words are beautifully sung:

'A long, long time ago . . .'

We join her in the chorus.

# Chapter Thirty-Six

❧

# A Book at Last

In June 2001, Emma sits her Psychology A-level exam and finds a place for herself on a foundation course in Art and Design at a local college.

She wants to be an art therapist, working with children and teenagers in trouble. Art Therapy being an MA course, she will need a degree, first of all, to be accepted on it. So, her life is taking shape. For the next four years Emma will be studying for two degrees, a BA and an MA, and will then go into a field of work which involves what she loves and what she is good at.

Her foundation year is rewarding, but also difficult. On the positive side she enjoys the course and the tutor, who recognises her artistic skills and talents. She is liked for the warm, friendly person she is, encouraged and applauded for her work – and, under these conditions, she thrives.

The difficult bit is her physical frailty. Along with an

increased difficulty in studying, her years of illness, her poor diet and little or no exercise from childhood have made her physically vulnerable. She is prone to sore throats, coughs, colds, stomach upsets and to feeling ill when she gets over-stretched.

But she has a big enough repertoire of being in life, of engaging with it, and enjoying herself, to survive these set-backs.

Having started her foundation course, Emma applies to universities and colleges outside London to do her first degree.

She has decided London, the city where she was born, is too big, noisy and impersonal and she wants to be a student somewhere smaller. Perhaps somewhere where she can escape to the countryside and the sea.

We talk during this time, about her leaving London, about her childhood, her relationship with Colleen, books she has enjoyed reading and about most things.

Neither of us has said out loud that a critical period of her illness is over. Neither have we spoken about the notes and diaries we have both kept, our individual versions of her journey through anorexia.

We do now. It seems safe, and I know Emma is keen to 'say something' publicly about her illness. She has talked, more than once, about anorexia being misunderstood. She thinks people at risk of suffering from it still have a romantic view of the illness, which is dangerous, and that older people, like parents, are in the dark.

Emma would like her journey to be recorded, to help others to realise what anorexia really is, and, also, to 'do something' with the pain she went through. There was so much of it. It would be good to make use of it, and not just put the diaries in a drawer, push them aside and forget.

She would like me to write a book, she suggests, about the long years of her journey through anorexia, as seen through her journals and mine.

Sitting at the table together at the end of a meal, discussing this, I ask if she remembers asking me, as a child, to write down the story of how we met in the pub, to put it in a book. Does she recall this?

Yes, she does.

What was it about?

Well, even though she was little, she must have known it was unusual, how we met. And it was very important to her to know me, to be in my house. And she knew I wrote books.

Emma's precise instructions, as an eight-year-old, were that I should write how we met, where we met, and all the things we did together so that other people could read about us. Her wishes have not changed that much.

By the spring of 2002 Emma has gained her place to study Art at a small college in a country town where she believes she will feel at home. Her phonecall on the journey back from the interview tells me she did really, *really* well. A few days later she receives a letter of acceptance. She is so excited and happy. And so am I.

One evening she comes over for me to do an interview with her, on tape, before she goes away. Although we have talked a great deal in the last few months, I need to be sure about certain things in order to write for publication. Anorexia, itself, for example, and the phrase, mentioned only once in her diaries about its 'hypnotic gaze'.

Emma says her illness *was* a kind of self-hypnosis which obliterated the outside world, a way of escaping life and reducing its proportions to what she could manage:

'I think not eating became a focus, and it blocked out everything else, my fears about living in the world: how do I do this and how do I do that? They were all wiped away by this huge need not to be eating.

'It was a way of escaping everything and I felt I could almost transcend things.'

I ask what feeling lies at the heart of anorexia.

'The word that comes into my head is oblivion. It offered me a choice to not have to think about anything, to be able to just switch off, and sometimes it was like I wasn't there, but that was what I wanted.

'I wanted to have nothing to think about, no worries, no anything because it all felt too much. The world felt like too much for me and I wanted to switch it off and the anorexia and bulimia offered me a chance to be able to do that.

'There's a definite feeling of superiority that goes along with it. It's a feeling of having risen above everybody else around you because you don't need food, you don't need anything to survive. And you feel Pure is the word.'

Emma does not use the word 'recovery' for this stage of her journey out of anorexia. She says that, because you choose this illness, once you decide to get better, you will:

'I never distinguished myself from the illness. I always felt it was part of me. I knew that anorexia is an illness, but at the same time I knew I was making a choice to be ill. I always knew that once I decided to get better, I would.'

The reasons for Emma's illness and for her decision to allow life in, rather than die, are intertwined and involve the beginnings of her feelings of belonging, of safety and of competence to be in the world.

Emma cites the structure of the Unit as being important to her decision to disengage from her illness, and the fact that she felt safe in it, and cared for.

'It was the first time I'd been in an environment where I felt comfortable with all the people around me. I felt "I can be here and I can talk to anybody" and that was something that had been missing from my life.'

She says her gradual move away from 'definitely wanting to die' to 'maybe wanting to live', to 'positively wanting' a life of her own was a slow process, in which therapy was very important:

'I did a lot of growing up. I learned more about life and a lot about myself. I learned to care for myself in small ways and get self-respect. I learned there wasn't anything terribly wrong with me, as I always thought there was.'

Talking about our time together, my visits to the Unit, Emma says:

'The happy times of my childhood were with you. And it helped that you knew my childhood.

'You knew what was happening in a way that all the therapists and people didn't because they weren't there. You were. You actually saw my childhood. You understood it.

'I remember you telling me in the Unit I wasn't a bad person. And that was important.

'And it was important for me to hear about life outside my little eating disorder world, hearing about the beautiful places in the world you talked about.'

When I ask why she pushed me away, when she was first becoming ill she says:

'I knew that you'd see. I knew you'd see there was something going on and you wouldn't be content to sit back and let it happen. Which is what I felt my parents were doing.

'And because it felt to me that my illness was something so important for me to be doing, I didn't want you to interfere. So I pulled away from you. I knew that if I let you, you would help me . . . and I wasn't ready.'

Emma talks of her illness as 'an escape from real life', which she wanted to get away from because she was so unhappy:

'I was a very lonely child and it's funny but the first word that comes to my head is "starved". I felt starved of affection, starved of love and I felt that it wasn't OK to ask for it. Maybe there was a sense that if I deserved it, it would be there. There must have been something I'd done which meant I didn't deserve it.'

In her growing up, Emma has come to understand, not only that she, herself, is not a bad person, but that neither is her mother:

'One thing I really appreciate about her is the way she brought me up to be open-minded, I feel grateful to my mum for that.

'I think I learned there was no point in fighting her any more, always wanting something to change. I thought "why am I fighting like this? Why don't I just accept her as she is?" And it's so much easier, because the truth is she won't change.'

About the issue of anorexia itself, and other people's experiences of it, especially those she was with on the Unit, she says:

'One of the common themes was definitely mothers, mothers who had a problem showing affection and love. And the other common thing, was childhood abuse, sexual abuse.'

And what about the fear of being fat when you are so thin, I ask her, and the sense of identity, of people with anorexia seeing themselves differently?

'A lot of the time when people with anorexia say they feel fat they're saying they feel something else.

'It's more "I feel wrong. There's something not right here and I don't know what it is but I'm going to call it "fat".

'It's more that you feel "bad". If you're thin, then having a mouthful of food doesn't suddenly make you fat.

'Pictures of thin women were something I'd latch on to

and think "Yeah, OK, this is how I want to look." But that was not the reason. It was an extra thing. If the magazines weren't there it would have been a girl in my class: "Yes, I want to look like her."

'For me it was about finding something that I *wasn't*, so that I had something to aspire to, because I felt like there was something wrong with me and I had to change it.

'I didn't know what it was that needed changing. So, thinness: "OK, I don't have that. If I have that I'll be all right."'

Emma remembers one incident very clearly in her journey from wanting to die to wishing to live:

'It was the smallest and the biggest change because in the last admission that I had in '98, when I'd been in for eight weeks, for the first few weeks I wasn't really going along with the programme at all.

'I was still feeling I really didn't want to get better and then one afternoon I was sitting in my room and some of the day-patients were out in the living room and I heard one of my friends, Julia, laughing.

'I realised it had been months since I'd laughed and that I wasn't getting any joy from life.

'It was almost like someone had let a bit of sunlight in and from that moment on I made a conscious decision to do things to help myself get better.'

The weeks before Emma goes away are busy ones for us both. As I prepare to begin writing – sketching outline chapters, rearranging notes – we talk about what she should buy to take with her, and about the exciting prospect of her new venture. One evening, she comes over with a bag containing all her diaries for me to read while she is away.

Touched by Emma's trust in me, by her willingness to hand them over, there is something else too, I believe, as she places a large plastic bag inside the door. She is glad to be rid of them into safe hands.

For they are heavy, as it turns out. Even with what we have been through, I am still unprepared for the weight, the despair of her illness, which returns to me through their pages.

Before she finally leaves for college, and her first experience of being a student living away from home, Emma has a party to celebrate her twenty-fourth birthday. She looks full, warm, happy and I realise how many friends she has gathered round her over these long years of hers, this complicated life.

# Chapter Thirty-Seven

੭ઠ

## OUT OF A GLASS DARKLY

The reason why people suffering from anorexia see themselves as normal size – or big – when they are actually a bunch of bones is because they are looking in a different glass which none of the rest of us can see.

Their internal mirror of self-identity is skewed. Their illness distorts reality and in it, through it, they see only their own 'badness' and the 'failure' of the world around them to provide what they need.

With the onset of clinical anorexia, they remove themselves from painful realities, and turn towards their other mirror-friend, the trance. Yet, in the main, it is the torment they wish to escape, rather than life itself, which is perhaps why they flirt with death when it comes close, not sure whether they want it or not.

Understanding a life is understanding its illnesses and Emma's illness has been eloquent in what it has said about the complex nature of anorexia and the mismatch, in her life, between what she needed and what she got. It is also eloquent in what it says about how she saw herself: what she found in her inner mirror of identity and self-appraisal.

For Emma's early sight of herself was in a dark mirror through which she saw herself darkly. From a young age, she thought of herself as 'ugly' and 'bad', which was then reflected outwards, into her behaviour and into the life which she led.

She had difficulties being accepted by other children. Adults, too, had a problem with her 'bad moods', frequent spells of 'feeling unwell' and persistent questions.

Experts view the mother's role, 'a maternal factor', as only part of anorexia, by no means present in all cases and, where it is, certainly not thought of as 'the mother's fault'. With Emma, however, there *is* something, not a fault, but a factor, and one of life's accidents.

I believe Emma's view of herself came from the absence of a certain kind of light, traditionally viewed as maternal, when a small child is 'bathed in the light of' her mother's smiling gaze.

This gaze, for Emma, was broken. She was only a baby – eighteen months – when her father left, and it would seem that the 'supply', the loving gaze of her mother, was switched off. A double 'desertion'. While many children would recover, Emma did not, and neither did Colleen.

It was visible, this lack of repair. Except for that one occasion, on a Welsh beach, I did not see Colleen delight in Emma, nor Emma bathed in her approval. On that after-noon off the Pembrokeshire coast, our clothes heading for Dover and Calais, it was different, Colleen's face reveal-ing the love she carried, switched off inside her, for her only child.

Emma's diaries show her problem with identity and how she secretly viewed herself. Not able to tolerate the badness inside her, she found a way of switching 'ugly' to 'thin' and 'bad' for the 'good' control over her riotous appetite which anorexia provided.
And the pay-off for this switch-over was a different mirror, the trance-like, hypnotic gaze of her illness.

However, this blotted out the world. It was a way of life. It *became* life, obliterating images and relections of other people, even those close to her. This further retarded her development, taking her away from experience and from the competence she needed in order to grow.

The fact that Emma was reticent, and had problems with other people's view of her, was clear from a young age.
I saw her, in a schoolyard, holding back and, when she did move forward, being awkward and too eager to please.

It is painful to watch a child who is not accepted by other children try and find her way in. *You* love her but that will not make up, either now, or in the future, for her sense of being kept out.

I also recall Emma's knapsack which was worn, summer and winter, on her back. I have a sense of its heaviness, not physically, but of the weight she carried on her shoulders, or in her heart, from a young age: a burden of unhappiness, guilt and 'badness'.

Of hope, too? Tenacity? For Emma tried to find what she needed, and, in small part, succeeded. She found a grown-up who would tell her stories, teach her to sing, play the piano and dance. So, she was resourceful, too.

A part of her turning her back on her 'best friend' is here, in her wish to know what life has to offer, to be fed story-food and to explore the rich landscape of her imagination.

'We used to curl up on your sofa together and you would tell me stories. That was very important to me.'

Beauty, too, is important to Emma and hurt her at one stage, making her weep, because it reminded her, I believe, of what she was not, and of what she could not bear to hold. In Crete, especially, the beauty of the mountains, the sea, the ordinary friendliness of local people, frightened her by so clearly demonstrating a reason to be part of life.

This at a time when she was not ready to make the journey out of her dark glass into the sunlight.

I have said at the beginning of this book that Emma's diaries were signposts pointing both ways. They were also trying to tell me, and herself, where she was. She was somewhere you would not wish to be: in the middle of a deeply confused, highly dangerous mess; an emotional maelstrom. It was not until I had read them many times that I began to see their pattern, fingerprints on a cave wall, her signals of distress.

My own non-expert experience of being with Emma leads me to call anorexia an 'emotional' illness. It was not physical in origin, for although its manifestation was through the body, as has been said, starvation and binge-eating are a person's *solution* to a problem, not the problem itself.

Nor, from where I was standing, is anorexia a mental illness, for I did not consider Emma to be paranoid or mad. She was, for the most part, in charge of her senses – but not of her emotions. These she was beset by, the size of them seeming to defeat her at times: anger; fear; despair; self-loathing.

Emma does not know the single cause of her malaise. Nor is there one. Of the many family doors and windows opening and closing in a child's house, who knows which let the problem in, or kept the answer to it out.

# Chapter Thirty-Eight

❧

## AUSTRALIA AND ADVENTURE

Returning from Christmas in Wales at the end of 2002 I find a message from Emma saying how nice it would be to see me. It will be the first time we meet since she left London in early October to go to college.

Her first term, which has ended a few weeks back, had been difficult and I have been thinking about her.

The first problem was the difference in age and in experience between her and other students. There was no one else she had met on her course who was older than eighteen or nineteen. They were nice and friendly, these other students, but it wasn't the same, being with people she felt so much older than.

Neither did Emma expect to have to be in an art studio every day for eight hours. Her artwork already advanced, she could do the work asked of her in a small amount of time and had to just 'be there' for the rest.

Her frustration was not helped by the other part of Emma's life, not socialising, as I had fondly thought, but earning money. To pay for her course and upkeep, she was working fifteen hours a week in a bookshop. Coupled with forty hours a week 'shut away' in a studio, there was not a lot of breathing space.

The news she brings when we see each other, ten days after Christmas, is that she has left college and is definitely not going back.

I am shocked. This is so final, and she had looked forward to going so much.

But Emma has only one plan now, to get a job – any will do – a flat with one of her friends who is back-packing round Australia at the moment and will be returning in the summer, and to enjoy earning some money, being with her friends and living in the Big City again.

Having left London, to her surprise she has missed it, she says, its broad-mindedness especially, which she has not appreciated till now. She had felt adrift at college, had missed her friends terribly and is ready to enjoy being back here, where she belongs.

But what about her MA?

'That can wait for now.'

But maybe it can't, I say. She is twenty-four. She might think of doing a part-time degree in London where she could be with her friends and study at the same time.

Emma seems to think this is a good idea.

Phoning her to see how things are going, she is really

excited. She is going to Australia, to join her friend who is out there for the last bit of her round-Australia trip. She hopes to go within a few weeks and will be back by the end of May.

I am really pleased for her. And then I ask about her plans for university.

Her voice changes. She is not going to do that for now.

Putting the phone down, I realise I am deeply disappointed and angry with this scenario, of Emma letting things which matter to her slip. Speaking to a friend, she sorts me out. It is marvellous Emma is going to Australia, she says. What a wonderful rite of passage. Just what she needs. For my part, I have done what I can, and should leave it to Emma. I must let her go.

So, over the next few weeks I keep quiet about the degree. Instead I say how glad I am she is making this trip, and sympathise with the delay over her visa. It arrives in the end and, in late February, an excited Emma rings from the airport.

She is on her way at last. Her first big adventure.

I do not believe Emma's love is unplaced any more. Nor do I think it is yet secure. She has a way to go. The postcard which arrives from Australia is vividly coloured and says she has seen amazing creatures of all hues: butterflies; pelicans; eagles; lorikeet; ibis.

'I'm having lots of adventures,' she writes, 'which you will hear all about on my return.'

The next one is in the same vein. She is thriving on sun,

fresh air, gorgeous beaches and is having a marvellous time:

'I look forward to seeing you when I return for a massive chat and photo session. Love, Emma.'

I know she has come to love life itself and to want to explore it at last, to go out and find what it might have to offer and to let it in. But Emma returns from Australia with Ross River Fever. Like malaria, it leaves her with little energy or appetite.

Slender, but seeming to be eating well enough when she first returns, her plans to get a job and move away from her parents' home are delayed, and become further delayed, as Emma begins to sink again. She finds the atmosphere at home difficult and takes to staying in bed and not eating.

Seeing her every few weeks, I do not notice the weightloss, first of all. Then, when she has been back for three months, the change is stark. Arriving to stay in my flat for a week while I am away, Emma has lost more than half a stone in a fortnight, possibly more, and looks anorexic.

I tell her so, straightforwardly, and she puts up little fight this time:

'No one else has told me I've lost weight,' is all she says.

On my return, she looks better, has been out looking for jobs and somewhere to live away from the 'home' that is, unfortunately, a dangerous place for her, and a reminder of anorexia's notorious persistence.

Packing away Emma's diaries, from where they have lain scattered round my desk, I notice, for the first time, the artwork on the cover of the plastic V&A bag they came in. On one side, two wrists decorated by Elizabethan ruffs lead to joined, but kid-gloved, hands. On the other side, a single hand in a black glove – a burglar perhaps? – holds an antique teapot, ready to pour, spout down. So, two renderings of a story, hers and mine.

What I found in Emma's diaries, eventually, after many readings, was a pattern among all the lava-flow, scratches in the rock, the route of her painful journey – not towards death, but away from somewhere she did not want to be.

I have no idea what Emma will do with her journals of anorexia. They may be read again, someday, or not. They may be best left in a deep drawer.

In handing them over to me, I believe she had wanted me to tame them as well as keep them safe and give them back to her in a more agreeable form. In taking heed of their riotous and romanticised emotions, she wanted me to transform them from thousands of distressed words into a story she can understand and live with: the book she has wanted since childhood.

Emma came from a sad, grey place. Not enough fun, warmth, colour, light. Now, she has found her way into a rainbow-coloured, adventurous life and I must let her lead it the way she chooses. Let her be.

She will meet the world, however she will, *her* way. And,

for my part, I give her these bundled-up words for her journey onwards:
the story of how we met;
a word-map of where she has come from.

# Chapter Thirty-Nine

## Expert Views

A dilemma for experts dealing with anorexia is that the journey out of the illness is highly individual and is not, therefore, predictable.

There is no 'anorexia pill' to be taken, or regime to be followed, which has a proven, consistent success rate. Research has come up with factors you might look out for in understanding patterns, where they exist. Within these, what Emma went through and what she 'presented' is not unusual.

Dr Adrienne Key, senior lecturer and honorary consultant psychiatrist at St George's Hospital Eating Disorders Service, in south London, told me:

'It's a very complicated disorder and we work with multi-aetiology, multi-factorial origins. That means there are various factors in the environment, in the personality and, possibly, in your genes.

'But I don't for one second think that anorexia occurs because you have an anorexic gene.'

She goes on to say: 'There's a strong link with personality traits like perfectionism.

'The other inherited traits are anxiety and what's called harm avoidance, a coping mechanism which draws people away from novelty.

'They retract [from novelty] and rather than being gung-ho about sorting out problems, their coping strategies tend to be to try and dumb down feelings rather than problem-solving.'

She concludes:

'It's a disorder in which there's a fundamental problem with self-identity.

'We're not absolutely sure what causes it, but we've got some good ideas. The things we do know is that it attacks young women [only 10 per cent of anorexics are male] going through very important developmental changes in adolescence and young adulthood and it occurs most frequently in western culture, or cultures exposed to western ideals on thinness and food excess.'

I notice Dr Key uses the word 'attack' for what happens with anorexia, and how easy it is to view the illness differently – as the sufferer's fault.

She works with mirrors in trying to bring about repair, asking women to stand in front of a mirror and tell her what feelings they have when they do so. She says:

'The outer mirror helps them to open the inner mirror

of identity. It helps them to access the problem – the lack of self-identity or a very negative self-identity.

'So the outer mirror helps to reveal the way we see ourselves, which is our internal mirror.'

Explaining why recovery takes such a long time, she adds:

'So much of the treatment comes down to helping an individual find out who she or he is.

'The illness attacks at a time of big developmental change in which you would expect to establish your self-identity, form relationships and develop from there.

'With anorexia, you have a big developmental break, which is very difficult to retrieve in all sorts of ways. It takes a long, long time.'

Dr Eric Johnson-Sabine, consultant in eating disorders and honorary senior lecturer at Royal Free and University College Medical School in north London, says he and his staff have around 5,000 attendances each year for people suffering from eating disorders, of which anorexia is one.

Like Dr Key, he views the illness as multi-causal, with high risk factors like weight concerns and perfectionism. Many factors are, however, individual, as are responses to treatment. He said:

'Different theories about anorexia ring true in some individuals, but everything doesn't ring true for everybody. That's why one tends to take what seems sensible from particular models. I don't think anything applies to all patients.'

What interests Dr Sabine is the large number of people who never come for treatment at all, but who live their lives with a degree of eating disorder:

'A lot of patients who are referred to us, by their GPs or other services, never come through the door. They don't keep their first appointment with us.

'Others come once and never come again. They're not so ill as to be brought here compulsorily, but they could be suffering. We feel these patients don't get the service, the help, we'd want them to have.'

Dr Sabine distinguishes between anorexia nervosa – or restricting anorexia – and bulimia nervosa, binge-purging, which he describes as far more common.

He says worldwide figures on anorexia in general show around 10 per cent of people dying from it. Another 25 per cent retain some level of anorexic eating disorder, and a further 15 per cent develop bulimia nervosa as an end-stage. This leaves only 50 per cent with no eating disorder after ten years of referral and treatment.

Not a good outcome – only a fifty–fifty chance of full disengagement with the illness – and one which reflects the bewildering and complex path which anorexia pursues.

The consultant in charge of the Unit where Emma received treatment describes her illness as fairly typical of how anorexia presents itself and the path it takes. He also speaks of Emma's journey as being at the severe end of the range of anorexic illness, and of Emma as being very ill indeed: because of the speed with which she lost weight;

and because of her low potassium level, which was life-threatening.

Emma's BMI was less than 13 and her periods stopped for six months and more a number of times over the acute part, almost five years, of her illness. Her medical reports, however, which she gave permission for me to see, reveal she was not considered suicidal.

What *was* unusual about Emma was the early onset of her illness in what is called a 'sub-clinical' form which was not life-threatening: the fact that she was raiding her mother's fridge from the age of eight while, at the same time, refusing the proper meals cooked for her.

When asked what parents and relatives should do about someone who is obviously not eating, who is losing weight, and possibly at risk of anorexia, the consultant gave the following guidelines:

1. Try and talk about it and, if you can, gain the teenager's co-operation. Introduce regular meals so that members of the family are not eating separately.

2. Agree on what these meals should consist of – and be consistent about what is expected. Especially, avoid battles, both between yourselves and with the person you are worried about. Present a firm front.

3. If you have co-operation from the person who is not eating, draw support from other people. Alert

teachers, and ask the school to supervise what is being eaten there.

However, he cautions, if battles start with the person who is not eating, then call in outside help straight away, either from a GP or by contacting the national Eating Disorders Association for a local contact. Once arguments develop, you need support from professionals.

So, a battle of wills will not win the war with anorexia. The path of Emma's illness showed this, that you cannot fight a person suffering from anorexia and expect to win. Their co-operation is needed if they are to wish to live their lives, and gain the means to do so, rather than retreat into the more 'reliable', less difficult, place of a trance.

This, in a sense, was the prize which Emma so wanted from anorexia, that she would substitute life's troubles and its unwieldiness for something else. Not death, but an easier state of being, one which did not frighten and challenge her so much.

And although, with Emma, magazines and images of thinness were not a spur to her illness, there is a message about thinness in western culture which links slenderness to being valued and to achieving ease. Thin woman are more prized.

Dr Key talks of advertising's contribution to anorexia in the following way:

'I think the bizarre contrast between hugely available amounts of food and an ideal of being thin is difficult for adolescents to manage.

'We are a culture of contradictions and this availability of consumer items and acquisition of money along with the absence of development of self must be a critical factor.'

# *Postscript*

*❧*

## KNOWING ANOREXIA

Emma's journey has given me an inside view of why people suffering from anorexia are so difficult to help. And with the low success rate even of specialist treatment for the illness, I have not seen the point, in this account, of making her path seem easier and more palatable than it was.

For a great part of the time I was with her, the girl I had known since childhood struggled with enormously bleak and destructive forces.

Emma's anguish, the complicated nature of her ambivalence, her wish to repeat her illness, and the variety of ages she presented and experienced at any one time are here, then, along with her unpossession. The latter took a long time to address and is important fully to appreciate for what it illustrates about other sufferers.

One doctor said he, himself, had discovered this lack when four patients came back from a trip to the supermarket empty-handed. They had literally not known what to do: how to shop; what amounts to ask for; and, importantly, how to decide between themselves what to put in the trolley, how to co-operate.

So, encouraging someone to relinquish anorexia is a complicated business. There would seem to be little point in returning someone to the outside world without the practical tools to survive. At the same time, as has been clearly said, a purely practical, 'let's get the weight back on' approach will not work.

I think it is possible to see anorexia as a 'replacement illness', as something which comes in, or is brought in, by a person suffering feelings which are too much to bear: both too much, and too little.

People with anorexia would seem determinedly to replace what is on offer with something of their own. For there is an emptiness in the middle of them which they wish to fill.

I was adopted as a replacement, a substitute for Colleen for a while, someone Emma could have an alternative relationship with. She needed me to see her through a different pair of eyes, ones which would see, and come to know, her better self.

All the more painful for me, therefore, was the possibility of her death.

My holding back from her at times lay in recognising and accepting this and my notes from visiting her contain many yearnings: 'Oh, dear Emma, I come away, longing, as I musn't, that you will live.'

While it is clear from talking to her and from a re-reading of her diaries that Emma did not want to die, she needed to exercise the right, to 'play with the power'.

The way I helped tip the balance was by refusing to 'get lost' in her dark glass. I did not collude with the hold her illness had over her. In part because it angered me and also because I had a way of spotting the difference between Emma and it. I knew her. She trusted I would remember who she was, even when she, herself, had almost forgotten.

Memory is crucial to identity, and when she was prepared to pick up her life again, it was invaluable to have someone there who knew what that life was.

To me, Emma's life, now, seems full of possibility, especially if she is alert to early warning signs of danger. Like her habit of using the phrase 'low energy' whenever she feels bad. It conceals what specifically might need to be looked at, I believe, masking possible depression and the beginnings of despair. In her strong moments, she says that anyone can get better from anor-exia – and I have to add the corollary, 'if they are vigilant'.

I have no difficulty understanding people's anger with anorexia and with its wilfulness, a child who wishes to die bringing the worse kind of despair for us all.

But what if the child does not want this, is saying, instead, that she or he has a tremendous problem with living? That, for whatever reason, whatever 'accident', big or small, being alive, finding a meaningful way in the world seems too much to accomplish? This is different and puts the problem, the bearing of pain, back into adult hands.

Emma was helped to move away from her illness through a long process, part accident and part design: the design of the Unit and of my story-food; the accident of a laugh from the next room.

The laugh, the stories, the safety, being cared for and being *known* reminded her of who and what she was missing. She began to want to live when the tug of big, surprising, unwieldy life became bigger than the downward pull of incompetence and despair.

In an acquisitive, speeded-up society, anorexia would seem to require more care, more patience, more attention to detail – in other words, more understanding – than most of us have the time to give. It asks difficult questions – beyond self-obsession – about relationships and how the connection between what is wanted and what is supplied is viewed: not only within families, but outside, in the world, which a person suffering from anorexia is afraid of:

What can be kept and ingested without guilt?
What is strengthening and of value?
What is alluring, but leads to the starvation of a dark glass?

People suffering from anorexia raise questions about what we imagine to be the nature and circumstances of accepting with ease and, especially, of belonging, and how we, as adults, pass on to children thoughts, feelings, attitudes about fulfilment. They ask questions, in a skewed world, about what is sustaining. Those who turn to the illness could be said to be in terror that the world will not recognise their emotional appetite and let them in.

I believe an attempt at a 'true story' like this has the power to let us in, to be insiders. To know, therefore, what it is like under the skin of the person something is happening to and to be compassionate. From the outside you have a wayward girl. From the inside you have a terrified one.

From my inside/outside view, I saw Emma's illness with a mixture of despair, anger and something she needed from me: both acknowledgement and refusal. My independence, if you like. She needed me not to collude with anorexia, but to know it on her behalf and to resist its shadowy beckonings and dark glass.

I have challenged Emma many times, something her mother has been unable to do because of their poor relationship. Yet, as someone gets older, challenging is more of a risk.

Years back, Emma wanted to be stopped and has in some measure found the means of achieving this for herself. She has moved from the anxiety of 'not enough' to the possibility of an inner home. She has sufficient balance and ease in the world to taste life, share it with others, place her love.

Emma has found she can take in food, experience and beauty from the world around her without pain or guilt and with this sustenance, she can continue to be strong. In her ease and belonging she will, I believe, have much to give in return.

# Afterword

## WRITTEN BY EMMA

I'll be starting my art therapy course later this year and I feel strong and happy.

When I look back on the person I was when I was ill, she seems like a part of me that maybe got lost. I don't feel any deep connection with her. I would say I recognise her, but there's no remaining familiarity. I see her as who I was, but I don't see her as who I am.

But she shaped the person I am today. She's given me depth and compassion. Without what I went through, I wouldn't have the insight I do. I'd be someone completely different now and I'd certainly be on a different career path.

Anorexia was a journey for me and it was something I needed to go through and was waiting to happen for a very long time before it did.

It's my belief that anyone can recover from anorexia.

Once I decided I would be better, I never doubted I would be.

But I wouldn't do it for anyone else. I wouldn't do it for doctors, for any of them. I knew when I was ready to I would do it for myself and it's my belief that anyone else can as well.

When I look back on the person I was then I think she just needed to be loved, to feel loved. If I met someone like her, I'd probably just give her a big hug. That would probably speak more to her than any words could.

Help and advice with eating disorders can be obtained from a family doctor, the following organisations, and further organisations linked through their websites:

The Eating Disorders Association (EDA) has a network of regional contacts. Send an SAE to:

Eating Disorders Association
Wensum House
103 Prince of Wales Road
Norwich NR1 1DW
helpline: 0845 634 1414
e-mail: www.edauk.com/shn.htm

The British Association of Psychotherapists
37 Mapesbury Road
London NW2 4HJ
phone: 0208 452 9823
e-mail: Mail@bap-psychotherapy.org

The British Psychoanalytical Society
112a Shirland Road
London W9 2EQ
phone: 0207 563 5000
e-mail: www.psychoanalysis.org.uk